The Atypical Mycobacteria and Human Mycobacteriosis

TOPICS IN INFECTIOUS DISEASE

Series Editors:

William B. Greenough III
Infectious Disease Division
The Johns Hopkins University
School of Medicine
Baltimore, Maryland

Thomas C. Merigan
Division of Infectious Disease
Stanford University Medical Center
Stanford, California

The Atypical Mycobacteria and Human Mycobacteriosis

John S. Chapman

A Continuation Order Plan is available for this series. A continuation order will bring delivery of each new volume immediately upon publication. Volumes are billed only upon actual shipment. For further information please contact the publisher.

The Atypical Mycobacteria and Human Mycobacteriosis

John S. Chapman

University of Texas Southwestern Medical School
Dallas, Texas

PLENUM MEDICAL BOOK COMPANY
New York and London

Library of Congress Cataloging in Publication Data

Chapman, John Stewart.
   The atypical mycobacteria and human mycobacteriosis.

   Bibliography: p.
   Includes index.
   1. Mycobacterial diseases. 2. Mycobacteria, Atypical. I. Title [DNLM: 1. Myco-
bacterium. 2. Mycobacterium infections. QW125 C466a]
RC116.M8C46   616.9'2   77-1824
ISBN 0-306-30997-1

© 1977 Plenum Publishing Corporation
227 West 17th Street, New York, N.Y. 10011

Plenum Medical Book Company is an imprint of Plenum Publishing Corporation

Printed in the United States of America

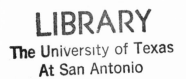

In Memory of
ANNE

Preface

Nearly twenty years ago a symposium convened at Dallas, Texas, to consider the place of atypical mycobacteria among agents of human disease. An edited and condensed version of that symposium was subsequently published and since that time has constituted the only bound source of information covering broad aspects of mycobacterial disease.

In the years since a vast amount of information has accumulated in periodical literature, some of which is not readily accessible. The time seems suitable for a comprehensive collection of this scattered material into a single book. The aim has not been to produce an exhaustive account of mycobacteria and mycobacterioses, but rather to concentrate on salient points and particularly on those most generally useful to a diverse group of interests: mycobacteriology, pathology, epidemiology, and, of course, clinical fields.

In Appendix A there appear in summary form manifestations of mycobacteria as they have occurred among clinical specialities, such as orthopedic surgery, dermatology, and urology. These summaries are designed to serve as guides to more probable infections and to lead to more extensive reading with respect to the specific organism encountered.

Appendix C presents, also in summary form, drugs, regimens, duration of treatment, and toxicities to permit ready reference to less familiar antimicrobial agents. These are suggestive only, useful when the general nature of the organism is known but not the specific susceptibility of the individual strain.

Interest in the atypical mycobacteria and their effects has been very lively during these past twenty years. Two decades ago infections caused by these organisms were something of medical curiosities. Reports at first dealt with all types under some general heading. A bit later it was sufficient to identify an organism as belonging to one of Runyon's groups. Since that time many organisms have achieved the status of species, some only quite recently. In consequence, both clinical and epidemiological reports have to be interpreted with respect to the time at which they appeared. Disease that is now recognized to be due to a particular species not long ago was identified only by group and before that only as an atypical mycobacteriosis, without differentiation.

Speciation even now is almost certainly incomplete. Classification remains unsettled. Appendix B, for example, demonstrates types of relationships among organisms that cut across and contradict the original schema of Runyon. Pigmentation and rate of growth are only two characteristics, and each may vary. In spite of this fact, it was decided to arrange material in this book according to Runyon's classification, primarily because it has become so familiar, but also because it remains a satisfactory point of departure for all but the most sophisticated.

Observation of and minor participation in this field of infectious disease, as it has developed during these two decades, has been vastly stimulating and rewarding. Association with many of the authors cited has surely been one of the most gratifying features of my life. I hope I have done justice to them and their work, and for any failures I apologize with great humility. To my own immediate associates in investigation I extend my hearty thanks.

John S. Chapman

Dallas

Contents

PART II. THE PHOTOCHROMOGENIC MYCOBACTERIA

PART III. THE SCOTOCHROMOGENIC MYCOBACTERIA

PART IV. THE NONPHOTOCHROMOGENIC MYCOBACTERIA

PART V. THE RAPIDLY GROWING MYCOBACTERIA

PART VI. APPENDIX

PART I

GENERAL CHARACTERISTICS

1

Early History of the Atypical Mycobacteria

Almost a hundred years ago Koch described the human strain of *Mycobacterium tuberculosis*. Within a short time, the bovine tubercle bacillus had been identified as a separate, specific organism, and within a few years, the avian mycobacterium had also been isolated and described. By 1895, not only were these organisms well known to bacteriologists, but in the course of their work, they had encountered many strains that did not coincide with descriptions of the original specific acid-fast bacilli. Investigators of the period undertook the same examinations of problems of origin, mutation, transmissibility, infectivity, and pathogenesis that their successors were to take up 50 years later. It will be evident from the account that follows that bacteriologists turned at once to the environment, not only as a source for the various strains but also as an intermediate habitat of tubercle bacilli.

I. ISOLATIONS FROM MILK PRODUCTS

Since milk obviously played a very important role in the infection of humans with *Mycobacterium bovis,* bacteriologists began to investigate that substance almost at once. By 1897, Rabinowitsch[298] had completed an extensive bacteriological survey of milk, butter, and other dairy products and had reached the conclusion that although these foods contained bovine tubercle bacilli, they also produced many other types of acid-fast bacilli. Among these was one organism that seemed to exhibit photochromogenicity.

Since milk products contained so many kinds of acid-fast bacilli, the question naturally arose whether these entered the milk from the animals' blood, from some ascending disease involving the udders, or whether they were simply contaminants unassociated with any infection in the animals. Rabinowitsch's work demonstrated that after careful disinfection of the udders, organisms were still present in a considerable proportion of specimens. These organisms, although they were acid-fast and microscopically similar to the tubercle bacillus, produced colonies that differed in rate of growth, in colonial morphology, and sometimes in pigmentation. To add to the problem of classification, some of these mycobacteria produced lesions in animals, while others failed to do so.[299]

Tobler, pursuing the work of Rabinowitsch, also succeeded in isolating many types of mycobacteria from butter and made one of the earliest attempts to classify them into groups according to their bacteriological and pathogenic characteristics.[381] Among pigmented colonies, she described one, similar to Moeller's Grass II, that seemed to exhibit a change of color as time passed, although she did not ascribe the chromogenicity specifically to exposure to light.

In 1903, so intensive had been bacteriological studies that Courmont and Potet[79] published a review of their own work and the studies of others. In this summary of organisms that had been isolated from many substances as well as from the environment, they found so many variations that any attempt at classification was impossible.

Almost all strains exhibited a remarkable vitality in their ability to grow on many kinds of media and at temperatures from 18° to 38°. At the higher of these temperatures, they grew rapidly, but it was in their capacity to form pigments that they were distinctive: "white or pale yellow in the beginning, they become golden or copper-colored or salmon with age. Besides temperatures, light and the composition of the medium often very much affect their chromogenicity." More than that, these investigators noted a difference in the capacity of these organisms to produce lesions or to elicit antibodies. In conclusion, they could not be certain that all these organisms were genuinely distinct from the tubercle bacillus, but as a practical matter, they had not resulted in important human disease.

II. ISOLATIONS FROM THE ENVIRONMENT

A fundamental question for all these investigators was not only if the tubercle bacillus might survive in the environment but where the organisms encountered in various milk products may have originated. Ward's study[413] demonstrated that milk at the time of secretion in the lacteals was sterile, but that it soon became contaminated as it traversed the ducts. Even before this observation, however, the concept that infection of animals might arise from the environment had led to extensive investigation. Moeller,[256] having already isolated and identified the timothy bacillus (*Mycobacterium phlei*), continued examination of cattle fodder and recovered a distinct acid-fast organism that he temporarily referred to as Grass bacillus II. Other bacteriological explorations of the barnyard resulted in recovery of acid-fast bacilli from the intestinal contents of animals, from both aged and recent manure, and from various kinds of feed, water, and soil.[80,256,257,260,299] It thus became evident that animals were continuously exposed to a wide variety of mycobacteria and harbored these organisms in their gastrointestinal tracts. There remained some possibility, not yet clarified, that these intestinal mycobacteria might produce disease or might enter the circulation and appear in secretions such as milk without actually having produced lesions in the host.

III. EARLY VETERINARY MYCOBACTERIOLOGY

Two sets of observations derived from studies in veterinary pathology continued to stimulate interest in atypical mycobacteria. The first of these, Perlsucht, a tuberculosislike disease of the omentum and mesenteric lymph nodes of cattle, produced a variety of mycobacteria that, for the want of any better terminology, were called paratuberculosis bacilli. Organisms isolated from the lesions in some instances could not be differentiated from some of the environmental organisms. Differential staining,[347] cultures at different temperatures, standard bacteriological techniques, and even immunological methods[346] failed to establish different identities.

Veterinary medicine had already established the existence of a specific infection of fowl by an identifiable species, *Mycobacterium avium*. That the organism's pathogenicity was not limited to avian life, however, was the subject of a 1908 report by Arloing,[8] who stated that bacteriologists had "found in tuberculous lesions of man, horse, mice, swine, monkeys and rabbits bacilli possessing the usual characteristics of the avian bacillus." Somewhat later, Meyer encountered very similar organisms in the mesenteric lymph nodes of cows. Upon intravenous injection, these organisms produced severe disease in young calves, but they failed to invade tissue if they were included in feed. He speculated nevertheless that transmission from cow to calf might take place through milk or that if sufficient contamination of pasturage took place, infection of very young calves might become possible. The characteristics of these organisms, as he described them, very closely resemble those now assigned to *Mycobacterium intracellulare*. In culture, they grew at 38° to form small, domed, white colonies, with little wrinkling. Injected into animals these mycobacteria produced sensitivity to Bang's avian tuberculin. Since injection of the bacilli into fowls, rabbits, or guinea pigs failed to produce gross lesions, Meyer concluded that organisms of this class might be regarded as occupying an intermediate position between *M. phlei* and *M. avium*.[252]

IV. ISOLATIONS FROM HUMAN MATERIAL

In 1899, Moeller reported recovery from humans of organisms very similar to those he had earlier isolated from the environment. Suspending plates of medium above the beds of patients in the sanatorium, he was able to recover acid-fast bacteria, especially if the sputum was thin or mixed with saliva. Colonies appeared in groups of two or three, but sometimes more. From his own nasal mucus, he was able to isolate acid-fast organisms on three separate occasions, and once, when he had bronchitis, he coughed up a small plug that contained mycobacteria that produced visible colonies in three or four days. He observed: "As my bronchial catarrh subsided, these bacilli also disappeared with it." A study of the nasal secretions of housemen and serving girls also produced mycobacteria on a number of occasions.[256,257] In conclusion, he regarded these atypical mycobacteria as perhaps normal or frequent contaminants of secretions of the upper airway: "In nose and throat mucus, on tongue and teeth, I have found these pseudo-tubercle bacilli."[258]

Of course Moeller's isolation did not establish more than human colonization, but in 1898, Pappenheim reported what seems to be the earliest proof of pathogenicity of atypical mycobacteria for humans.[279] He observed a young woman whose illness resembled gangrene of the lung. During her illness, he isolated from sputum and after her death recovered from severely infected pulmonary tissue an organism that he could not specifically identify but that possessed many of the characteristics of *Mycobacterium smegmatis*. Dieterlen likewise recovered from the sputum of a patient with pulmonary disease an organism that grew in colonies of an "orange bis gelbroter Farbe."[97] Though this patient did not react to tuberculin, the organism upon injection into animals produced occasional, limited, caseating lesions.

V. A LATENT PERIOD IN MYCOBACTERIOLOGY

After the initial enthusiasm generated by the extensive investigations at the turn of the century, interest in mycobacteria waned. From the "practical" point of view, there were two kinds of organisms that produced human disease, *M. bovis* and *M. tuberculosis*. All other mycobacteria were saprophytes. In the United States, and probably elsewhere, laboratories ceased engaging in cultures for mycobacteria or, if they continued occasional bacteriological investigation, threw out cultures the colonies of which they regarded as atypical, and hence, probably, contaminants. If an unusual organism occasionally appeared, the court of last appeal was injection into guinea pigs and rabbits. If the organism failed to produce progressive disease in either of these two species, it simply had no interest.

But also this was the epoch of the rise of sanatoriums, most of which were staffed by young physicians who had entered the field because they had acquired tuberculosis in the period of their training. In consequence, they lacked both bacteriological skill and the necessary energy to carry on much extensive investigation. Among the established laboratories, such as the Phipps in Philadelphia, the laboratory at Trudeau, and the Pasteur in Paris, attention turned to the production of more purified types of tuberculins, analysis of the components of the tubercle bacillus, and search for effective means of vaccination. Finally, the intervention of outside events—World War I, a period of wild inflation in Europe, and total economic disaster in 1929—necessarily impaired the ability of laboratories to carry on research.

In spite of these various obstacles, a few laboratories continued to engage in careful mycobacteriology, to search for new organisms, and to try to arrange them into logical order. Beaven and Bayne-Jones, for example, report an illness in a child of 11 weeks of age. There was extensive disease of the lung associated with pleural effusion. From the pleural fluid, the investigators recovered an organism that produced abundant colonies in seven days. Growth was much delayed at 22°. The acid-fast bacillus did not reduce nitrate and produced only a faint tinge of yellow pigment. Though the infant did not respond to tuberculin, she did manifest delayed hypersensitivity to an antigen prepared from the isolated mycobacterium. After a long time, the disease underwent resolution and eventuated in calcification.[18] The authors were convinced that they had witnessed the equivalent of primary tuberculosis as a result of infection with a ''nonpathogenic'' mycobacterium.

Max Pinner, almost alone, continued the type of investigation that had proved so fruitful 30 years earlier. By 1932, he had isolated a sufficient number of strains of organisms from pulmonary disease in humans to lead him to propose a classification. Of particular interest are his Groups II and III. Strains characteristic of Group II produced smooth, white, easily dispersed colonies; organisms produced only local ulcers in guinea pigs. Pinner's Group III organisms included 11 strains, all from human material. The bacilli themselves appeared microscopically to be larger and more beaded than human tubercle bacilli. All strains in this group produced a lemon-yellow or orange pigment and, upon injection into animals, resulted in tubercle or abscess, usually localized.[289]

In a subsequent paper, Pinner extended his observations on both types of atypical organisms. The pigmented group had been isolated not only from human material but also from tap water, from nasal secretions, and in seven instances from urine. These resembled his previous Group III in pigment and in consistency. In animals, they resulted in a few noncaseating tubercles, but on serial passage virulence increased. Importantly, the investigator observed that injection of these organisms, regardless of the extent of lesion, induced allergy to tuberculin in guinea pigs.[290] The problem of the Group II organisms was somewhat clouded by the fact that by careful picking Pinner was able to secure consistently smooth colonies of *M. tuberculosis*.[291]

Expanding on Pinner's limited immunological investigation, Wenkle, Loomis, and Jarboe examined problems of immunity in animals that had received injections of Pinner's Group III, pigmented organisms. These animals exhibited cross-reactions both cutaneously and serologically against the antigens of *M. tuberculosis*. But in addition, these investigators showed that preliminary injection of these organisms protected animals against subsequent challenge with viable *M. tuberculosis*.[426]

VI. HUMAN INFECTION BY AVIAN OR AVIANLIKE MYCOBACTERIA

In 1908, Duvall isolated from the cervical lymph node of a young Canadian woman an acid-fast organism pathogenic for fowl. After a short period of progressive ill health, the patient developed an overwhelming and fatal miliary disease. Post mortem examination revealed miliary tubercles involving all the internal organs. Histological examination revealed characteristic miliary tubercles, and cultures demonstrated great numbers of mycobacteria in all these lesions. Duvall's description of the cultures leaves some doubt as to the exact nature of the organisms, in that in cultures held for a very long time he was able to find occasional small patches of red pigment against the "wax-like whiteness" of the colonies. What is important is the demonstrated pathogenicity for fowls and the fact that this early there is a documented and thoroughly studied case of disseminated infection caused by an organism other than *M. tuberculosis,* an organism that almost certainly would now be considered a member of the avian-Battey complex.[103]

While beyond any doubt, bovine tubercle bacilli produced disease in human hosts, it was not established that avian organisms might also produce disease in man. Crawford (1938) argued that even though definite evidence was lacking, human infection with *M. avium* might be expected.[81] Infection of chickens was very prevalent in the north central United States, he argued, 80% of tested flocks having presented evidence of infection. The organism was proved to have produced disease in sheep and swine, evidence that it could invade mammalian species. If hens were infected, their eggs also contained avian tubercle bacilli,[349] and in consequence a route of infection existed. Only the uncertain question of some kind of transformation of the organism might make its identification difficult.

Veterinary studies had thus laid the predicate for recognition of avian tuberculosis in man, and in 1943 Feldman and his associates[121] reported the case of a miner with silicotuberculosis whose sputums repeatedly produced in pure culture an organism that required two weeks of incubation for the earliest colonies to appear. The colonies were "nonchromogenic" and dysgonic. The family were all negative to mammalian tuberculin, but the organism was not pathogenic for chickens. However, it did produce cross-reactions with *M. avium* both in skin tests and serological examinations. The authors concluded that the mycobacterium represented some intermediate between *M. avium* and *M. tuberculosis*.

In 1949, Dragsted[101] reported the isolation of similar organisms. In Denmark, since 1935 there had been six cases of human infection. Two children less than 4 years old had cervical lymphadenitis caused by these organisms, and similar strains had been isolated from the axillary lymph nodes of a 15-year-old girl and from epicondylar and axillary nodes of a 24-year-old woman. Organisms of the same type, hardly distinguishable from *M. avium,* had grown out of the spinal fluid of a 5-year-old child with meningitis and from the sputum of a middle-aged male who had apical infiltration and fibrosis. All these organisms differed from *M. avium* only in the lack of pathogenicity for chickens.[101]

In the same year as Dragsted, Feldman *et al.* reported the case of a 22-month-old child with massive lower-lobe pneumonia. Bronchoscopic aspiration of sputum produced acid-fast mycobacteria that seemed to be either *M. avium* or a very nearly related organism. Epidemiological investigation of the environment established that 50% of the chickens, two of the six swine, and 30% of the cows on the farm where the child lived reacted positively to avian tuberculin.[122]

VII. EPIDEMIOLOGICAL EVIDENCE FOR "SAPROPHYTIC" INFECTION OF HUMANS

Throughout the 1950s, Palmer and his associates had carried out extensive studies of human sensitivity to PPD. Their most striking finding was the prevalence of numerous small reactions to this antigen, as well as a considerable group of young people who failed to react to the 5-TU dose but who did react to the 250-TU dose. Furthermore, they were able to show that this low-grade sensitivity to PPD had a characteristic distribution, being greatest in the southeastern United States and lowest in the northwest.[105,276]

In 1961, D. T. Smith *et al.* furnished what appeared to be a partial explanation of low-grade sensitivity in the southeast. They demonstrated that students from that area reacted rather strongly to avian tuberculin, although their reactions to PPD were weak or absent. The studies of both groups made it seem probable that human infection—or perhaps more accurately, sensitization—had occurred through contact with mycobacteria other than *M. tuberculosis*. Until more specific antigens might be developed and applied, however, more specific statement was impossible.[339]

Underlying theory in these early epidemiological studies was the premise that a group of individuals should react to a homologous antigen with a "normal" or Gaussian distribution of responses. Whatever the antigen, there were always excessive numbers of reactions in the range of 2–6 mm, and the unavoidable inference was that still other mycobacteria might have produced the abnormal distribution.

The work of MacCallum and associates[233] in Australia in 1948 supported such a possibility, for they reported a specific ulcerative disease of the skin developed from infection with a hitherto unknown but highly specific mycobacterium. Freeman had also isolated from a patient with multiple subcutaneous abscesses an organism that closely resembled *Mycobacterium fortuitum*.[128] The earlier findings of Pinner, moreover, made it seem possible that in special situations, almost any kind of a mycobacterium might invade human tissue and produce a disease characterized by the formation of tubercles.

VIII. CLASSIFICATION

The general view of mycobacteriologists by 1950 held that there were the familiar three varieties or species of *M. tuberculosis:* human, avian, and bovine. In addition to these, there were several species of well-known "saprophytic" organisms: *M. phlei, M. fortuitum,* and possibly *Mycobacterium butyricum.* However, Pinner had already established the existence of other organisms occasionally pathogenic for man and had attempted a classification. Gordon's classification of 1937[141] was that of a bacteriologist. Saprophytic mycobacteria could be arranged in an order or a set of groups, according to pigmentation, colonial morphology, carbohydrate utilization, effect on litmus milk, requirements for glycerol, and dependence on specific temperatures for optimal propagation. Out of 252 strains, she found that 80% could be classified into three groups, with two subdivisions in both the second and the third groups. Her classification indeed was a bacteriologist's refinement of that already proposed by Pinner. Two characteristics of these earlier classifications led to their early neglect: they were couched in the technical language of bacteriology, and they did not pertain to a subject that clinicians regarded as important. Tobie's attempt at classification in 1948 achieved no better acceptance.[380]

During the decade after World War II, however, partly at the instance of the Veterans Administration, clinical laboratories throughout the nation began to culture sputums routinely. With increasing numbers of cultures came new problems both for the directors of laboratories and for clinicians. Even the mistaken classification of the organism by Cuttino and McCabe[84] as *Nocardia intracellulare* served as an impetus to mycobacterial classification.

Isolations of mycobacteria that had to be regarded as atypical (with respect to *M. tuberculosis*) had become so frequent as to result in confusion both in the laboratory and on the ward. By 1954, Timpe and Runyon elaborated a system of classification that suited the needs of the time. It is given in full in Table 1-1. The genius of this classification lies in its

TABLE 1-1
The Timpe–Runyon Classification[a]

Group	Pigment	Rate of growth[b]	Colonial features
I	Photochromogenic	14–21 days	Rough, eugonic
II	Scotochromogenic[c]	10–14 days	Smooth, eugonic
III	Nonphotochromogenic[d]	14–21 days	Dysgonic
IV	Variable	5–7 days[e]	Eugonic

[a]For other classifications, see Appendix A.
[b]Rates of growth are those usually given. New isolates from human material may require a longer time, and strains repeatedly subcultured may grow much more rapidly.
[c]As cultures age, many of them darken from yellow to deep orange and exhibit small patches of red pigment.
[d]The term allows for a few strains that exhibit light yellow or lemon-colored pigment that is not affected by exposure to light.
[e]The short time required for full-growth accounts for the alternate use of *rapid growers* as a designation for this group.

separation of slowly growing from rapidly growing organisms and in its division of the slowly growing organisms according to the very simple and readily understood character of chromogenicity. Its acceptance and success have stemmed from its simplicity and applicability to clinical problems.[377]

At the time the classification was offered, it seemed that pathogenicity for humans was limited to Groups I and III, but it soon became apparent that some strains of Group II and Group IV might also occasionally invade human hosts. Various modifications have already occurred, and unquestionably further modification will become necessary. But the effort of Timpe and Runyon merely to group organisms rather than to speciate them produced a system sufficiently elastic to allow modifications without disruption of the classification as a whole.

IX. ORIGIN OF THE ATYPICAL MYCOBACTERIA

For at least the first half century after the discovery and identification of the human tubercle bacillus, it was regarded as the "type" organism of all mycobacteria. Its supposedly central position arose not only from its overwhelming preponderance as a human pathogen but also perhaps from an unconscious anthropocentric view of nature. Any mycobacterium that differed significantly from the type was by definition "atypical." This attitude made very little difference until it became certain that some of these atypical forms were pathogenic for humans. There was the further fact that the human bacillus produced lethal disease in guinea pigs, whereas these other organisms resulted in only local lesions. The implied conclusion was that man should be more rather than less resistant than a guinea pig to any type of mycobacterium.

As recently as 1961 and 1965, authorities have argued that atypical mycobacteria are in fact only variants or dissociants of the tubercle bacillus.[304,439] Various modifications in media are known to affect the appearance of colonies of *M. tuberculosis*.[260] Since the atypical mycobacteria had been isolated from a variety of different environments, the possibility existed that all these strains might represent some type of resting or vegetative forms that would revert to normal appearance after a certain period of residence in the human host. Straus and Dubarry, for example, had shown that mycobacteria might survive for protracted periods in sterile water and lose neither viability nor pathogenicity.[357] In the view of one writer, subsequent changes in characteristics might be more closely related to the host than to the organism itself,[260] and even avian and bovine species might represent variants of the human organism. As early as 1908, Theobald Smith addressed this problem[343] but could only conclude that while such transformation was possible, there was no adequate evidence to prove that it occurred.

Another line of evidence entered into the argument that the atypical organisms represented mutations from *M. tuberculosis*. It had been observed that now and again patients who had far-advanced tuberculosis, having become sputum-negative, after a time began to expectorate material that contained numbers of scotochromogenic organisms totally resistant to all drugs. These, it was argued,[304,439] represented mutations induced by isoniazid, PAS, and streptomycin.

Finally, dissociation of mycobacteria had been known for quite some time. It had been shown to occur with respect to both *M. tuberculosis* and other organisms.[352,353] If such dissociants occurred spontaneously, it would seem theoretically possible that similar variants might occur within a human host. (It is hardly necessary to observe that bacterial genetics at the time of some of this discussion was practically nonexistent.)

Since the majority of authors no longer adhere to the belief that atypical mycobacteria represent only specially selected mutants of *M. tuberculosis,* a summary of the evidence for their opinion follows:

1. Atypical organisms were isolated from the environment as far back as 1895, and isolations from human material occurred almost as early; isolation from diseased human tissue took place frequently before 1948.

2. The use of PAS and streptomycin was very infrequent before 1948, and isoniazid did not come into use until 1952. Therefore, drug resistance and mutations induced by these substances could not have occurred earlier.

3. Some of the atypical mycobacteria have a specific geographic distribution, a characteristic that seems to identify them as being environmental organisms only accidentally pathogenic for man. This distribution does not accord with drug-induced mutation.

4. Genetic mutations, when they occur, characteristically involve an enzyme system, and only one, whereas as the discussion of the bacteriology of these organisms will demonstrate, species differ extensively.

5. The opportunities for isolation and identification of these organisms have increased enormously by reason of the widespread use of cultures.

6. The epidemic of human tuberculosis has been waning at least since 1900, and therefore the frequency of isolation of atypical mycobacteria in relation to isolations of *M. tuberculosis* has undergone a very marked increase.

7. There has never been adequate demonstration of transformation of *M. tuberculosis* into any atypical mycobacterium.

8. When mycobacteria are subjected to Adansonian classification, *M. tuberculosis* no longer occupies a central position[386] but, as Wayne stated the situation, appears in a "very peripheral position, where its sharply limited distribution in nature suggests it belongs."[417] In short, *M. tuberculosis* represents one of a genus of Mycobacteriaceae; it is specifically selected for parasitism for mammals, especially for man, and fails to survive for more than a few minutes outside a host.

2

Bacteriology

Discussion in this chapter deals with general studies of bacteriological and antigenic properties of the atypical bacteria. Specific traits within groups, as they apply to identification, will appear in discussion of individual organisms.

I. CULTURAL CHARACTERISTICS

A. Media

All mycobacteria grow well on media ordinarily employed for *M. tuberculosis:* Loewenstein—Jensen, Petragnani, Long's liquid medium, Sauton's liquid or solid medium, 7H9 and 7H1O. (This statement does not refer to *M. bovis,* with its special requirements for glycerol.) Possibly simpler media would also support the growth of many species. There has been little study of minimal requirements, though Kazda[188] established that "moorland" water (standing water in small pools) provides sufficient nutrients to permit the multiplication of Group III organisms.

Distinctive features of *M. fortuitum* consist of its ability to grow on cornmeal agar and on oleic-acid agar medium, while *Mycobacterium xenopi* produces characteristic branching, filamentous forms on cornmeal medium.[155]

B. Rate of Growth

Whereas *M. tuberculosis* requires 6–8 weeks for growth on the standard media, primary isolates of Group I and of Group III organisms usually
achieve complete growth in 21–28 days, and Group II organisms normally
attain mature growth in 10–14 days. Members of Group IV require as little
as 4 or 5 days, though if their origin is human tissue, a slightly longer time
may be required. (These rates of growth represent average figures for
primary isolations. Organisms that have been subcultured repeatedly require much less time. Isolations from human material, particularly if some
form of antimycobacterial therapy has been employed, may require considerably longer.)

C. Oxygen and CO_2 Requirements

Atypical mycobacteria appear to be obligate aerobes, with adequate
gas tensions provided by loosely closed screw caps. There has been no
concerted search for anaerobic mycobacteria, but certainly none of the
usual strains tolerates much under 10% oxygen. Some appear to grow
better at CO_2 concentrations of 5%.

Wayne and Doubek have established that the photochromogenicity of
Mycobacterium kansasii is dependent upon an adequate oxygen environment, as well as upon exposure to light during the phase of rapid growth.[419]

D. Temperature Requirements

Mycobacterium marinum requires incubator temperatures of 27–28°,
while *Mycobacterium ulcerans* grows best at 32–33°. Strains of true *M.
avium* call for temperatures of 45°, as apparently do some strains called *M.
intracellulare*.[396] However, it is possible that some of these strains of
intracellulare would now be classed as *M. xenopi*,[100] which characteristically calls for higher temperatures. (Statements with respect to requirements of temperature relate especially to primary isolations; organisms that
have been carried through numerous subcultures may adapt to different
temperatures.)

E. Hydrogen Ion Concentration

Steenken and Smith have reported long since that nonpathogenic variants suffered greater injury from NaOH than from H_2SO_4[353] and found that most of these strains grew better at pH 6.2 than at pH 7.2. The usual descriptions of atypical mycobacteria pertain to the appearance of cultures grown at pH 7.2–7.6. However, it has been shown that characteristic strains tolerate a wide range of pH,[50] organisms of Group III in general displaying ability to grow at from pH 3.6 to pH 9.8. Other atypical mycobacteria could reproduce at narrower ranges, while *M. tuberculosis* displayed the least tolerance. The final pH of the liquid medium was only slightly altered at termination of growth. Kazda's study of *M. intracellulare*, strain Davis,[188] confirmed that that strain tolerated a low pH.

F. Colonial Morphology and Pigmentation

Colonial characteristics are described more fully under the section dealing with the individual mycobacterium. Pigmentation constitutes the basis for the first three groups of Runyon. Photochromogenicity results from exposure to light during the phase of rapid growth, but this is not an absolute quality since both scotochromogenic and nonchromogenic strains of *M. kansasii* are known.[312,366] Dependence upon oxygen for formation of pigment has already been mentioned. Hydrogen ion concentration[50] affects production of the pigment, as well as the incorporation in the media of drugs to which the organisms are partially susceptible.

In the case of *Mycobacterium szulgai,* photochromogenicity is affected by temperature, for the organism is scotochromogenic at 37°,[327] while at 25° it is photochromogenic. *Mycobacterium simiae* is reported to possess only weak photochromogenicity, but this information is based on cultures maintained at 37°,[202] and variance from that point might reveal a difference.

All Group II organisms produce a strong yellow pigment when cultured with complete exclusion of light. As cultures age and exposure to light is repeated, the pigment deepens to strong orange, and very small flecks of red pigment may be observed against the background.[192]

The pigments produced both by photochromogenic and scotochromogenic organisms appear to produce identical absorbency spectra in the ultraviolet, in the expected region of carotenoids. If *M. kansasii* is extracted before exposure to light has resulted in production of pigment, absorbency is similar to that of nonchromogenic organisms or *M. fortuitum*.[354]

Pigment among Runyon's Group IV organisms varies with the species. Those of clinical importance, *M. fortuitum* and *Mycobacterium chelonei,* do not form pigment.

G. Cording and Orientation

The formation of serpentine cording in cover-slip preparations is characteristic of *M. tuberculosis* and may be apparent in as few as 12 days.[231] Richmond and Cummings, however, reported that a somewhat similar cording might be observed in cultures of *M. phlei* and of the "radish bacillus" (*Mycobacterium terrae*).[309] Very loose and incomplete cording of *M. kansasii* has also been observed in our laboratory when a cover-slip preparation was employed. In subcultures of various mycobacteria, Gilkerson *et al.*[136] reported the finding of distinctive microcolonial features in as short a time as 96 hours. With some of the reservations indicated, authorities generally hold that in liquid cultures atypical mycobacteria show no cording and are random in orientation.

II. BIOCHEMICAL ACTIVITY

A. The Niacin Test

This examination, which tests the ability of organisms to synthesize niacin, has proved the single most valuable method of excluding *M. tuberculosis* from the possibilities offered by an unknown organism. Konno found this ability almost invariably in strains of *M. tuberculosis,* while in 132 strains of atypical mycobacteria, he encountered none that formed niacin.[199] Subsequent wide employment of the test has served only to confirm its reliability; the only exception is the recently identified *M. simiae,* which is identifiable otherwise by its photochromogenic pigment.

B. Catalase Production

Early studies indicated that when *M. tuberculosis* became resistant to high concentrations of isoniazid, it also displayed a loss of catalase. With the decline in production of catalase, there was a diminished pathogenicity for animals. Most members of Groups I, II, and IV produce vigorous catalase reactions, while pathogenic strains of Group III produce the enzyme only in small amounts. (See Tables 2-1 to 2-4.)

Wayne has modified the original test by studies of catalase activity after subjecting organisms to heat at 68° and by differentiating in a semiquantitative fashion between organisms that produce a column of foam of greater or less than 45 mm.[418] Andrejew and Gernez-Rieux[6] attempted to differentiate the structure of mycobacterial catalases by the use of various inhibitors, but the steps were complicated and neither classification nor differentiation was much improved. Similar recent studies of the active substance have examined both molecular weights[150] and methods of enhancement and inhibition[95] but have not yet reached the point at which extensive interspecies comparisons are available.

C. Tween Hydrolysis

In 1948, Dubos and Middlebrook observed changes in pH as a result of growth of *M. tuberculosis* in a medium that contained Tween 80[102] and

TABLE 2-1
Distinguishing Features of Photochromogenic
Mycobacteria[a]

Feature	Organism		
	kansasii	*marinum*	*simiae*
Growth at 37°	Yes	*No*[b]	Yes
Niacin production	No	No	*Yes*
Nitrate reduction	*Yes*	No	No
Tween hydrolysis	Yes	Yes	*No*

[a]In this and all succeeding tables those tests that have no differential value *within the group* have been omitted.
[b]Deviation from features of other organisms indicated by emphasis.

TABLE 2-2
Distinguishing Features of Scotochromogenic Mycobacteria

| Feature | Organism | | | |
| | Pathogenic | | Nonpathogenic | |
	scrofulaceum	szulgai[a]	gordonae	flavescens
Nitrate reduction	No	Yes	No	Yes
Catalase hi	Yes	Yes	Yes	Yes
Tween 3-day	No	16–49%	Yes	Yes
5% NaCl	No	No	No	Yes
Urease	Yes	?	No	Yes

[a]This organism is scotochromogenic at 37°; photochromogenic at 25°. The most common differential is between *M. scrofulaceum* and *Mycobacterium gordonae* or *M. flavescens*, in which the 3-day Tween hydrolysis would be the critical distinction.

proposed that neutral red be incorporated as the indicator in the test, which they hoped would serve to separate pathogenic from nonpathogenic organisms. Hydrolysis of the wetting agent releases oleic acid, and the test has been applied particularly to differentiation among types of Group II and Group III organisms. With rate exceptions failure of a strain to produce hydrolysis points to pathogenicity.[333,421] (Wayne advocated both a three-day and a seven-day reading.[421])

D. Nitrate Reductase

Virtanen[408] reported that *M. tuberculosis* very strongly reduces nitrate to nitrite but that reductases of *M. bovis* and *M. avium* are weak and slow-acting. Among atypical mycobacteria, *M. kansasii*, *M. szulgai*, and all Group IV organisms except *M. chelonei*[34,420] produce vigorous nitrate reductases.

E. Amidases

In 1960, Bönicke applied a series of amide-splitting tests to a number of strains of *M. kansasii*[33] and found that the strains were entirely consis-

TABLE 2-3
Distinguishing Features of Nonchromogenic Mycobacteria

Test	Pathogenic			Nonpathogenic		
	avium	xenopi	ulcerans	gastri	terrae	triviale
Nitrate	No	No	No	No	Yes	Yes
Cat. h̄i	No	No	Yes	No	Yes	Yes
Cat. 68°	Yes	Yes	No	No	Yes	Yes
Pigment	No	Yes	No	No	No	No
Tween	No	No	No	Yes	Yes	Yes
Tellur.	M[a]	No	?	No	No	No
5% NaCl	No	No	?	No	No	Yes
Arylsul.	No	M	No	No	No	F[b]
Urease	No	No	No	Yes	No	No

[a]50–84% of strains.
[b]16–49% of strains.

tent in their possession of amidases. In extension of his earlier work, he then proposed a series of amide-splitting tests as a means of differentiating among species of atypical mycobacteria. Japanese and European investigators have employed these measures to a much greater degree than Americans, who have usually limited their studies to urease activity only.[205,207,418] The possession of a strong urease is especially characteristic

TABLE 2-4
Distinguishing Features of Group IV Organisms

Test	Pathogenic		Nonpathogenic		
	fortuitum	abscessus	phlei	smegmatis	vaccae
Niacin	No	Var[a]	No	No	No
Nitrate	Yes	No	Yes	Yes	Yes
Pigment	No	No	Yes	No	Var
Photo pigment	No	No	No	No	Yes
Tween	M[b]	No	Yes	Yes	Yes
Iron uptake	Yes	No	Yes	Yes	Yes
Arylsul.	Yes	Yes	No	No	No
MacConkey	Yes	Yes	No	No	No
Urease	Yes	Yes	No	No	No

[a]Variable.
[b]50–84% of strains.

of *Mycobacterium scrofulaceum, M. fortuitum,* and *M. chelonei* (see Tables 2-1 to 2-4).

F. Arylsulfatase

Tests for the presence of this enzyme have been extensively employed in the United States. Except for *M. xenopi* and some strains of *Mycobacterium triviale,* the presence and activity of this enzyme are a characteristic of Group IV organisms.[208] Readings should be made at the end of 72 hours.

G. Reduction of Tellurite

This test is of particular value in identifying pathogenic strains of the avium-Battey complex from nonpathogens. Unfortunately, the results are not common to all isolates and should be correlated with a negative Tween 80 test. The incorporation of tellurite in solid media results in somewhat different results from those indicated in the tables. A recent study of selenium salts in solid media provides somewhat the same information but may provide a better differentiation among Group III organisms.[354]

H. Other Biochemical Tests

Tests for the presence and activity of lipases and galactosidase,[370] heat-stable phosphatase,[317] and production of acid phosphatase; ability to utilize various inorganic sources of nitrogen,[385] utilization of specific compounds as a source of carbon;[387] and tolerance of and effects upon a series of inorganic salts of metals[58,354] have all been examined in a search for simpler or more certain techniques for identification of atypical mycobacterial. The results thus far have produced no generally practicable techniques.

I. Mycobacterial Resistance

Resistance to isoniazid and streptomycin is a prominent feature of many atypical mycobacteria. The characteristic is not constant, however, and as discussion of susceptibility of various organisms will make evident, resistance to antimicrobial agents is not universal with respect either to organisms or to drugs.

Tests are commonly carried out in liquid subcultures with drugs at varying concentrations, which may be the range from the lowest bacteriostatic concentration to the highest attainable in the patient. This has been the technique most often employed in research, while in many laboratories, for clinical purposes, direct sensitivity on plates containing 7H10 medium has been the method of choice. One quadrant serves as control, while the other three characteristically have contained streptomycin, PAS, and INH at midconcentrations. Results of the two different methods are fairly consistent, provided inocula contain approximately the same numbers of well-dispersed organisms.

The last proviso is most important, as the work of Canetti,[42] and Wichelhausen and Robinson[427] has established. Among other points, it was demonstrated unmistakably that inoculation of mycobacteria in small clumps might produce a wholly misleading result with respect to streptomycin. Furthermore, if inocula are quite heavy, important aspects of susceptibility will surely be overlooked.

It should be understood that resistance is an all-or-none genetic feature of a clone of organisms. Since cultures of wild strains contain many clones, it is far more accurate to speak of a certain percentage of organisms as susceptible than to employ the much less informative statement that 2-plus growth occurred at 5 μg/ml. By the far more accurate (and more difficult) method advocated, a comparable examination of susceptibility at 5 μg/ml might show a control growth of 100 colonies, with only 20 colonies on the drug-containing medium. It is obvious that this method leads to a far different concept, that is, that 80% of the organisms are susceptible. It should be evident that the numbers of organisms inoculated in control and in each of the drug-containing media must be as nearly as possible identical. It is also obvious that solid media with light inoculations permit a far more accurate appraisal of the potential effects of an antimicrobial agent.

In spite of the relative crudeness, however, one can expect to obtain perceptible effect from the use of a drug that reduces a 4-plus growth to a 2-plus growth, but the effect will be brief unless one or more other antimicrobials of similar effect are used. (At the recommended dosage of the various antimycobacterial drugs, one can expect to achieve peak concentrations in human serum at least as high as 5 μg/ml.)

Resistance to drugs and various chemicals has been the subject of numerous reports: these include susceptibility to salicylate,[452] to p-nitrobenzoic acid,[130,400] to nitroxiline,[374] to triphenyltetrazolium,[155] to erythromycin,[261] to rifampin,[316,390] and to cycloserine.[163]

J. Adansonian Classification

All the studies cited above have been intended to result in the clarification of relationships among strains within species and the establishment of distinctions between species. In some instances, work has not been repeated. The bits of information are so numerous and in some cases so special that investigators have sought means of reducing the number of tests and increasing the specificity of their identification. Some of the most troublesome areas of differential diagnosis occur among the many varieties of Group III and among some organisms of Group II that lie in an uncertain area[192] between Group II and Group III.

As bits of information multiplied, comparisons between species and between strains became increasingly complex, and a purely statistical method of classification and identification has evolved, the Adansonian method. This method avoids the bias of selection of one test or group of tests as ''better'' or ''more informative'' than another and gives the same weight to each characteristic. By this method, an unknown strain may then be carried through a battery of tests and the results compared on a statistical basis with tests of what is regarded as a standard organism. Similarly, numerous strains of what appear to be the same organism may be subjected to the battery of tests, and from the average results of tests in all strains, a ''hypothetical mean organism'' may be constructed.[32,205,372]

For example, out of 95 different tests, one Japanese investigator selected 59 that seemed to possess differential utility, 29 for slow-growing (Groups I, II, and III) organisms, and 34 for rapid-growing organisms (Group IV).[388] In America, Kestle et al.[192] employed studies of 47 characters and, after applying them to a series of strains of the same species, produced what they termed a ''median reaction pattern'' for the species as a whole. An unknown would be identified as a member of the species if it attained a comparative score of 90% similarity.[386]

For well-equipped mycobacteriological laboratories, not designed for intensive research, it was obviously necessary to reduce the tests and simplify the procedures by which an unknown mycobacterium might be identified with a reasonable degree of accuracy. This applied particularly to strains and subgroups within Groups II and III. Leading American authorities now recommend the tests included in Tables 2-1 through 2-4 as being satisfactory for use in good laboratories and probably adequate for purposes short of research.[205,207] (In the original publication, all these tests were included in a single, inclusive table.)

III. CHEMICAL STUDIES

In addition to biochemical studies of metabolic activity, it is possible to analyze the organisms themselves for evidence of specific materials. Smith and co-workers[340,341,342] undertook analyses of organisms for specific lipids and identified by infrared spectroscopy a number of mycosides that appeared to be specific. Within Group II, they found three categorizing mycosides, as well as glycolipid apparently specific to *M. kansasii*. Lipid components among Group III organisms, however, were very heterogeneous.

In a related area, Reiner *et al.*[305] applied pyrolysis and gas–liquid chromatography to reveal what they regarded as "finger-print" regions specific to various organisms. In their opinion, the materials they studied consisted of components of the cell wall.

Marks and Szulga employed thin-layer chromatography for examination of lipids among strains of *M. fortuitum*. Among their 17 strains, 4 clearly departed widely from the patterns of their type strain (Cruz.). (At the time of this experiment there was considerable confusion as to the place of *Mycobacterium abscessus* and *M. chelonei*.[245])

IV. PHYSICAL METHODS

Lethality of ultraviolet light for mycobacteria has been the subject of a study[89] that demonstrated greatest susceptibility in *M. tuberculosis* and least in *Mycobacterium flavescens*. The authors concluded that resistance was directly proportional to the production of pigment. Susceptibility to irradiation from a Co source has been examined as a means of assaying survival[23] and mutability. Susceptibility of organisms to heat has been mentioned in Chapter 1 and will be more fully detailed in Chapter 3. Group III organisms seem to have an unusual capacity to withstand higher temperatures.

V. BIOLOGICAL METHODS

The tuberculin test itself constituted the earliest recognition that *M. tuberculosis* contained antigenic materials, and as has been shown in the preceding chapter, early identification of human infection by "saprophytes" led to the production of various kinds of testing materials. During the first half of this century, most researchers engaged in studies of antigenic components of the tubercle bacillus for two highly pragmatic purposes: to produce some sort of nonliving immunogenic agent and to devise some kind of laboratory test that might assist them in deciding upon the clinical activity of disease. Though all these efforts produced a considerable body of knowledge of the chemical constitution of *M. tuberculosis* and though immunogenic substances have been found in cell wall, nuclear material, and various chemically extractable components of whole organisms, all efforts failed in the accomplishment of the two main purposes. Nor have studies of the antigenic components of *M. tuberculosis* ceased, though the complexity of the problem seems to be constantly increasing. Wright and Roberts,[437] for example, using two-dimensional electrophoresis, have demonstrated the presence of 36 precipitable antigens in the tubercle bacillus, rather more than Kniker[196] found several years ago by a different mode of separation. However, comparisons between results are affected by the great variety of methods of preparation of antigens,[52,59] as well as by the several modes of separation and the reactions employed to identify the antigenic substances.

A. Bacteriophage Typing

For a time, identification of organisms by specific lysis by bacteriophage seemed to offer considerable promise. Mankiewicz's study employed phages isolated from human stools against *M. tuberculosis*,[238,239] but Cater and Redmond isolated mycobacteriophages from soil and stockyards in an effort to obtain material adaptable to the study of atypical mycobacteria.[46] In this undertaking, they were only partially successful: they obtained fairly good adaptation of a phage of *M. kansasii* but less than satisfactory results with respect to the avium-Battey complex. The subsequent work of Kubin *et al*.[209] provides an explanation: they found no member of the complex susceptible to any of the phages they employed.

B. Hemagglutination

In 1955 Decroix *et al*.[93] attempted use of a crude polysaccharide fraction of *Mycobacterium tuberculosis* in an immunological study of patients who failed to react to tuberculin. Since then, Daniel and his associates[85,86,87] have been able to obtain highly purified polysaccharides for use in the hemagglutination method of Boyden. Some of these appear to be highly specific to strains of atypical mycobacteria. While this undertaking may prove too difficult for clinical application, it should provide important basic information.

C. Precipitins

Diffusion of antigens against antibodies in an agar gel system after the method of Ouchterlony[272] seemed to offer an excellent possibility of identifying strains with great accuracy as well as of determining relationships among species and subspecies. Parlett and Youmans[280] quite early undertook to apply the technique to the study of atypical mycobacteria, employing human sera against antigens. Subsequently,[281] they applied the same methods, using sera of specifically immunized animals. Among the pathogenic atypical mycobacteria, they found troublesome cross-reacting antibodies, though the method served quite well to exclude nonpathogens of the Runyon groups. Nor did any modification serve well when the technique was extended to human sera.[282] The same difficulties appeared in the studies of Rheins *et al*.[306] and of Burrell and his associates.[41] Other investigators, attracted by the apparent relative simplicity of the technique, attempted refinements by variations in the mode of production of antigens, in concentrations of antigen and antibody, and in the pH of the gel of the diffusing substances[4,238,376] without materially improving results. However, Lind[226] and Lind and Norlin[227] developed highly successful techniques and employed diffusion in agar with excellent results in the classification of some organisms. Likewise, the work of Stanford and Beck produced excellent results in their study of species.[350] In the author's laboratory, studies of human serum against antigens of atypical mycobacteria and *M. tuberculosis* proved useful as a means of excluding the tubercle bacillus as the cause of lymphadenitis in children[30] but could not be extended to study of sera of adults with pulmonary mycobacteriosis.

D. Agglutinins and Agglutinin Absorption

As early as 1948, Wenkle *et al.*[426] employed agglutination as a means of study of ''chromogenic acid-fast bacilli'' isolated from human material. Disparity between dermal and serological reactions, as well as troublesome cross-reaction with antigens of *M. tuberculosis,* interfered with the extension of their studies. By the early 1960s, however, Schaefer[324] succeeded in producing potent antisera and developed an absorption technique that has proved to be highly repeatable and invaluable in producing order among members of Groups II and III. A combined study of bacteriological methods as opposed to phage-typing and to agglutination[167] established that Schaefer's methods produced results identical with those of bacteriology with respect to *M. kansasii* and with less than 1.0% difference in identifications of Group III organisms. Phage-typing resulted in about 1.0% error with respect to *M. kansasii.*

Acceptance of Schaefer's work has been general.[313,418] As will appear in Chapter 3, agglutination and agglutinin absorption place Group III organisms from soil in distinct serotypes and have enabled investigators to determine sources of infection with far greater precision. However, the technique has proved itself particularly with respect to pathogenic organisms of Group III. *Mycobacterium xenopi,* previously regarded as a somewhat aberrant strain of Group III, was recognized as a distinct species through Adansonian classification; serological studies have confirmed and established this speciation, as they have rejected the speciation of *Mycobacterium brunense*.[211]

Application of agglutination reactions to Group IV organisms has been equally rewarding. Excellent agreement between lipid chromatography and this serological test[175] has resulted in reclassification of *Mycobacterium borstelense* as a strain of *M. fortuitum* rather than a species, as Adansonian analysis seemed to require.[389]

With respect to Group II organisms, results have also been very satisfactory. Bel[21] compared biochemical and bacteriological properties with agglutination in a study of 51 strains of *M. scrofulaceum* isolated from lymph nodes. Of these strains, 48 produced amidases in accord with Bönicke's spectrum D, the other 3 with spectrum A or C. Serological studies established 41 strains as *M. scrofulaceum,* while 4 corresponded with serotype Lunning and 4 with serotype Gause, and only 2 were untypable. Adansonian analysis established that serotypes Lunning and Gause are varieties of *Mycobacterium aquae nonurealyticum,* unique among organisms from lymph nodes in possession of a Tween hydrolase and a heat-stable enzyme that splits phenyphthalein dibutyrate. In this study, since both "Lunning" and "Gause" originated in infected human nodes, serotyping provided more exact information than the amidase series.

E. Other Methods

Other biological tests for identification of atypical mycobacteria have included such measures as sensitization of animals followed by a battery of skin tests,[234,315] challenge after induction of sensitization,[277] and rates of recovery of viable units from viscera of infected mice.[399] None of these methods has resulted in improved precision of mycobacterial identification, and many of them have not been tested by other investigators.

3

Epidemiology

Chapter 1, on the history of the mycobacteria, has made it evident that mycobacteria are present in soil, water, and feed for animals. Contamination of human foodstuffs, eggs, milk, and milk products had been established, and it was well known that these organisms infected or colonized many hosts. In the interval between discovery of these acid-fast bacteria and 1940, bacteriologists had also established their infection and colonization of humans.

These facts, reinforced by studies that followed, failed to establish a route of infection of humans. Known isolations had established that infection or colonization might occur through the respiratory tract, through the gastrointestinal tract, or—but presumably quite rarely—through inoculation. Organisms might reach a human host through aerosolization from soil, plants, or water; they might theoretically be transmitted directly from animals to man, or they might reach a human host indirectly through ingested substances such as water, meat, eggs, milk, and milk derivatives. The possibility of direct human-to-human transmission, as in other airborne infections, also had to be considered.

Such was the theoretical situation when interest in the mycobacteria once again developed. At first, reports consisted primarily of frequency of isolations in the laboratory. Reports of this type were inclusive of all atypical organisms, but after the acceptance of Runyon's classification, they became detailed with respect to the group to which the organisms belonged. Within another five years, sufficient information had accumulated and conditions for a clinical diagnosis had sufficiently matured for studies to limit themselves to frequency of disease, in contrast to rates of isolation in the laboratory. Finally, with an increasing precision of identification, a far more exact epidemiology, relating to species and identifiable strains, has developed.

During this period of increasing precision, and perhaps on the basis of analogy with tuberculosis and histoplasmosis, it seemed that skin tests with specific antigens might help to delineate the extent to which human exposure had occurred and, if geographic variation was a factor, to determine the nature of the limiting factors. This chapter, then, deals with a more general epidemiology of atypical mycobacteria and efforts to clarify epidemiology by means of skin testing, while the later and more specific epidemiology of particular organisms appears in the chapters devoted to each.

I. SOURCES IN THE ENVIRONMENT

A. Soil

Isolations from soil and water appear very early in the history of the atypical mycobacteria, primarily as by-products of a search for *M. tuberculosis* at some place in the environment. As these organisms attracted renewed interest, investigators again turned to these same sources in an attempt to learn the source of human infection, and from samples of soil, mud, and standing water, many strains of Groups II, III, and IV have been isolated.[48,187,206] In a more precise recent study, Tsukamura and his colleagues sought for and identified specific serotypes of *M. intracellulare* in the dusts of the rooms of patients with mycobacterial pulmonary disease. However, they found that organisms excreted by their patients were of serotypes entirely different from those recovered from the floors of their rooms.[393] Their results deserve emphasis from two standpoints. First, they suggest that patients produce relatively slight contamination of their environment, at least so far as the settling out of organisms is concerned.

Second, they establish that the flora of a room does not readily result in colonization even of an individual with previous disease of the lung.

B. Water

Isolations of mycobacteria from water had occurred toward the end of the 19th century. As early as 1889, Straus and Dubarry[357] demonstrated that mycobacteria might survive for weeks in either sterile distilled water or in sterilized pond water, with diminished rates of survival as temperatures were progressively increased to 37°. Since 1950, mycobacteria have been repeatedly isolated from water available to animals.[187,188,237,269,373,379]

These references include findings in many parts of the world and indicate that mycobacterial contamination of outside pools and standing water is very common. Gruft *et al.*[149] have even demonstrated the presence of strains of *M. intracellulare* in the spray and foam of ocean water, and Kazda[188] has added the final necessary demonstration that "moorland water" contains sufficient nutrients to permit multiplication under natural conditions.

More recently, attention has turned toward tap water as supplied by ordinary urban distribution systems. These studies developed because numerous efforts to isolate *M. kansasii* from other environmental sources had been nonproductive. From tap water, Bullin and co-workers[40] isolated strains of *M. xenopi;* Goslee and Wolinsky[142] recovered from tap water in Cleveland *Mycobacterium gordonae* as the most frequent isolate, but they also identified a number of other strains, which they place in an uncertain zone between *M. scrofulaceum* and the avium-Battey complex. In France, Tison and associates[379] recovered *M. kansasii* once from a large number of samples, together with many strains of *Mycobacterium aquae* (presumably *M. gordonae*). Gruft[148] isolated from tap water in America a number of strains of *M. kansasii* that differed from type strains in that they possessed only weak catalase activity. However, from tap water in California Bailey and associates[11] at last isolated strains of *M. kansasii* with characteristic high catalase activity. In addition, they showed that these strains might be isolated from taps in one distribution system but not from a nearby system with a different source of supply. If other studies result in similar findings, the sharply limited distribution of mycobacteriosis caused by *M. kansasii,* as observed, for example, in Czechoslovakia,[269] will be adequately explained.

II. HUMAN FOODSTUFFS

As related in Chapter 1, some of the earliest investigations, stimulated by obvious concern for human infections resulting from *M. bovis,* turned to milk and secondary products. More recently Tacquet *et al.*[369] isolated *M. aquae, M. avium,* and 10 unclassified scotochromogenic organisms from sediment of commercially centrifuged milk. Harrington and Karlson's study,[160] to the extent that pasteurization could be simulated in the laboratory, proved that strains of atypical mycobacteria, particularly those of the avium-Battey complex, could survive exposure to pasteurizing heat. Subsequently, it was reported[57] that milk subjected to standard commercial "flash" pasteurization and packaging contained mycobacteria of the same complex.

Eggs had been found to contain *M. avium* after hens had been infected with that organism,[349] and meat also was found to contain atypical mycobacteria,[378] although apparently infection was confined to lymph nodes most of the time. The strains isolated by Kubin and co-workers from animals of Czechoslovakia, however, were found to be varieties of the "Davis" strain, in Europe one of the less common isolates from human material.[211]

III. MYCOBACTERIOSIS OF ANIMALS

The importance of *M. bovis* as a human pathogen led very early to examination of the carcasses and viscera of animals for evidence of disease. As a technique for the detection of infected animals, the tuberculin test began to be applied in veterinary medicine almost as soon as in human medicine. Subsequently, an avian tuberculin was developed for examination of chickens and other domestic fowl. The eradication program in the United States and the quarantine programs adopted in Europe very soon encountered problems of reactors that, on examination after sacrifice, revealed no gross lesions (the "N-G-L reactor"). Since on many farms cattle, swine, and chickens shared the same environment and a common space and might have access to a common source of feed and water, investigators rather quickly entertained the possibility that *M. avium* might be a sensitizing organism among mammals as well as being pathogenic for birds. In 1938, Crawford[81] was successful in culturing avian organisms from chickens, swine, and even sheep. Stadnichenko *et al.* obtained similar results from sheep and swine slaughtered in the stockyards of Chicago.[348] Using the skin test with avian antigen as the measure of infection, Feldman and his colleagues[122] found evidence of parasitism by *M. avium* of cattle, chickens, and swine. With increasingly exact methods of identification, Tammemagi and Simmons[373] were able to show that *M. intracellulare,* serotype VI, could be traced from feed and water to sensitized and infected pigs and chickens, and Kazda[187] similarly traced *M. brunense* (now serotype "Davis") from pools of standing water to chickens. In Japan, isolations from swine were identified as serotype "Davis,"[394] the same strain identified under similar conditions in Czechoslovakia.[211]

The Mallmans and their colleagues previously had shown that sensitivity to avian antigen was widespread among pigs in the north central United States,[236,237] but they had also established that lesions might or might not be present. In France, Tacquet *et al.*[368] had similar experiences, as did Green[144] in England. The problem extended even to horses, as Konyha and Kreier showed.[200] In summary, the results of all these studies demonstrated that reactions to sensitins could occur in the absence of lesions or positive cultures; organisms might be recovered from normal tissues, or lesions might be limited to lymph nodes. On the other hand, it was also common experience to discover lesions or to obtain positive cultures from animals that failed to respond to sensitins.

Studies of anthropoids failed to produce resolutions of these difficulties. Karassova and co-workers,[185] for example, found tuberculin reactors in almost 50% of a colony of *Macacus.* Upon sacrifice and painstaking cultural study, 9 monkeys' tissues produced *M. simiae,* 4 produced strains of Group II, and 16 bodies yielded strains of Group III. From bodies of *Macacus* in their native habitat, however, Weiszfeiler *et al.*[425] isolated only *M. simiae.* From all of this, it is evident that in birds and mammals, including anthropoids, the discriminatory ability of sensitins is relatively poor in particular animals, however useful the skin test may be when applied to populations.

IV. SKIN TESTING IN HUMANS

Several bits of evidence seemed to suggest that applications of mycobacterial sensitins to human populations might clarify the extent and distribution of infections. Histoplasmin, as Furcolow had demonstrated only a few years earlier, had delineated an area of high prevalence of that fungus. Tuberculin (or PPD) had also been extremely useful in human populations as a measure of total exposure and also as a means of tracing infection in contacts. In spite of the variable and unpredictable results veterinarians had encountered in various species, antigenic substances prepared from atypical mycobacteria offered promise of clarifying a number of points with respect to the epidemiology of these infections among a human population.

It had already been shown that young people who were lifetime residents of certain regions of the United States exhibited exceptional numbers of small reactions (< 6 mm) to PPD intermediate and that the employment of second-strength PPD resulted in a reaction rate approaching 70%, a figure entirely disproportionate to the known rate of disease in the area from which they came.[106,267] Furthermore, the distribution of these excessive numbers of small reactors was clearly determined by some kind of geographic determinant, as had been the situation with respect to histoplasmin. In the case of PPD, the highest rate was in residents of the Gulf Coastal states and the lowest in residents of the Northwest.[276] On the basis of expected specificity, investigators then began preparation of PPDs from atypical mycobacteria, following the procedures for production of purified proteins from *M. tuberculosis*.

Extensive skin testing followed. In the southeastern United States, PPD-B (prepared from a strain of *M. intracellulare* isolated from a patient's sputum in the Georgia State Hospital) produced results that seemed to explain the unduly high proportion of small reactions to PPD-S (as the investigators called the derivative of *M. tuberculosis* they employed as a standard).[106,276] However, PPD-B elicited a disproportionate number of small reactions also, and the distribution of sizes of reaction assumed a bimodal rather than the expected Gaussian curve. When other sensitins (PPD-G, obtained from the Gause strain of scotochromogenic organisms; PPD-Y, produced from a strain of *M. kansasii*) were employed, the same deviation from the "normal" distribution was observed.[104] Tests with these and several other preparations in the Phillipines and in India[105] and even in Georgia[71] led to confusing results. In 1960, Nissen-Meyer[267] concluded that "PPD-B is a less specific antigen, or it has a wider antigenic spectrum, than PPD-S." Comstock[71] came to the conclusion that purified protein derivatives of atypical mycobacteria failed to provide an adequate answer: "To our perplexity and surprise, the mean sensitivity of the group tested in 1950 was considerably less than in 1952."

As additional tests were carried out in other areas, deficiencies of the mycobacterial sensitins became increasingly evident. In Chicago, where *M. kansasii* was remarkable for its prevalence, Pfuetze et al.[286] compared PPD-S with PPD-Y in patients with known disease and found that they reacted with complete crossover; that is, patients with mycobacteriosis kansasii reacted to PPD-S as well as to PPD-Y, and patients with proven tuberculosis reacted to PPD-Y as well as to PPD-S. At Duke, Smith and co-workers[339] noted striking changes in the patterns of reactions to sensitins among students and concluded that some kind of nonspecific mycobacterial sensitization was widespread in that area. However, when Smith and Johnston specifically sensitized guinea pigs and tested for reactions, they encountered even in such special preparations extensive cross-reactions between avian sensitins and those of Battey and of scotochromogenic organisms.[338]

Taking a somewhat different approach, the Dallas group,[53,219,294] using a tuberculin prepared from two strains of *M. kansasii,* found that of 201 children who were household contacts of patients with pulmonary mycobacteriosis kansasii, around 40% responded to the homologous antigen with reactions of 6 mm or more. Only 22% of children not in contact with "open" cases responded with reactions of the same size.[17] It was noticed, however, that rate and size of reaction increased with age between 6 and 12 years.[53] When the same group of exposed children were retested with the same material during the next 12–18 months, however, it was observed that about one-third had increased the size of reaction, one-third had decreased (in two cases becoming nonreactive), and about one-third had remained the same.

A similar variation in size of response to O.T. was observed among a group of noncontact children who had originally come to attention because of reaction to a multiple puncture test. Subsequently, Grzybowski and associates in Vancouver[153] came to the conclusion after extensive testing that in the area about 25% of reactions to PPD of between 10 mm and 14 mm were in fact nonspecific and probably resulted from other mycobacterial sensitization, while if the reactions were between 5.0 and 9.0 mm, 50% were the result of heterologous sensitization. In another special study, an effort to improve the specificity of the skin tests through the use of protoplasmic fractions of the organisms failed to improve results.[215]

When these materials were tested in Norway, Bjerkedal could not discover an antigen that appeared to account adequately for reactions,[29] and Magnusson et al.[235] had similar experience when they applied these mycobacterial PPDs to young Dutch males. In a very different setting (South India), Wijsmuller and associates,[429] after noting progressively larger reactions to PPD-G as the age of children increased, concluded that "low-grade sensitivity to tuberculin PPD-S is caused by a group of nontuberculous mycobacteria rather than by a single species" and that all of these organisms were antigenically somewhat closer to the Gause strain of *M. gordonae* than to *M. tuberculosis*. Finally, in 1974, Wijsmuller and Erickson[428] disposed of the specificity that once was thought to be a feature of PPD-B in the following words: "the vast majority did not acquire their sensitivity to PPD-Battey through infections with *M. intracellulare*."

While Americans had followed these lines of investigation, striving persistently toward greater specificity and a larger number of sensitins, elsewhere, and particularly in the United Kingdom, epidemiologists concentrated on a single antigen derived from *M. avium*. As far back as 1943, Jensen and Lind[177] had employed avian tuberculin as a general test for sensitivity induced by atypical mycobacteria. Though Beck and associates reported in 1962[20] that a similar avian antigen had failed to discriminate among infected swine, Kane and Vandivere[184] reported excellent specificity in guinea pigs. In Europe, at any rate, as subsequent serotyping was to show, the choice of an avian antigen was most fortunate, since it has now been demonstrated that Avian I and Avian II account for most nontuberculous mycobacteriosis that has been identified.[27,326] Skin tests in children in the United Kingdom, for example, have demonstrated a high rate of reaction to an avian sensitin, and sensitization by avian or avianlike organisms seemed to be the best explanation of aberrant tuberculin reactions.

As study continued, however, and as the same children were retested with the same antigen, the observations that had been made with a sensitin of *M. kansasii* were confirmed: "The acquired tuberculin sensitivity was temporary and tended to be lost or greatly reduced over a period of two years." The committee of the Medical Research Council continued[451]: "Over the follow-up period of two years the size of the reactions to the two PPD's avian and human decreased, particularly in the first six months. The size of the avian reaction decreased more rapidly than the human. . . . The control children who had been nonreactive before acquired a similar amount of both human and avian sensitivity" similar to that of the original reactive group. In a word, sensitivity to atypical mycobacterial antigens was not a fixed and repeatable response, as in tuberculosis, histoplasmosis, or coccidioidomycosis.

Further evidence to support this view came from a study of Judson and Feldman,[181] who performed tests with a *marinum* sensitin on a group of people who earlier had suffered infection of the skin and from some of whose lesions the organisms had been isolated. When tested 12 years after the infection, 18 of 44 former patients produced reactions less than 10 mm, and 10 of the patients responded with less than 5 mm of induration. The importance of this report is that in these people the organism was known to have invaded tissue and to have produced a chronic infection.

From the foregoing account of experience with skin tests, several important points emerge:

1. Mycobacteria possess very similar antigens, so that differential tests for hypersensitivity have very little discriminatory power.

2. Upon retests of the same individual, there is evidence of waxing and waning of response. When populations are retested after an interval, some have acquired and some have lost hypersensitivity as measured by available sensitins.

3. There seems to be a fairly constant rate among populations of the same age, with evidence that the rate gradually increases through childhood.

4. All sensitins that have been tested so far result in a bimodal distribution of sizes of responses.

The study of Robakiewicz and Grzybowski[310] especially underscored the problem of a constant rate in a population, a finding common to all the earlier studies. It should be obvious that if acquired hypersensitivity to mycobacteria is of long duration, similar to that of *M. tuberculosis, Histoplasma capsulatum,* or *Coccidioides immitis,* the rate of reaction should increase steadily throughout life. If the rate does not increase, the only explanation possible is that people lose hypersensitivity rather readily. The difference between tuberculosis, histoplasmosis, and coccidioidomycosis, on the one hand, and these mycobacterial conditions, on the other, is that in all of the first three, there exists a readily demonstrable invasion of tissue with spread to draining nodes, a feature that will be shown to be almost unknown with respect to mycobacteria other than tuberculosis. The inference must be that for most individuals, contact with the atypical mycobacteria occurs as colonization rather than an invasion and that from the immunological point of view, the situation more nearly parallels colonization with *Candida* or *Aspergillus* than invasion by a pathogen.

If acquisition and loss of hypersensitivity occurs as readily as the Medical Research Council report suggests, bimodal distribution at a given moment may be the result of small reactions associated with either recent gain or recent loss of hypersensitivity, as portions of a population acquire or get rid of a mycobacterial flora. It is possible, of course, that the sensitins employed have resulted from an unlucky decision. The recent elegant study of Chase and Kawata[59] reveals how readily one may impair a significant antigen in the course of preparation of a substance to be used for skin testing. It is possible that in deciding to follow the same methods employed for production of PPD-S, the originators of the atypical PPDs may have impaired the most important antigens of their preparations.

V. SEROLOGICAL STUDIES

Reference to serotyping of the "Davis" strain of *M. intracellulare* has already appeared. This type of examination has resulted in far more accurate information with respect to specific pathways through nature to a host than any previous undertaking. In these infections, as Lesslie and Zorawski[220] demonstrated in guinea pigs, an inverse relationship exists between skin test and serological antibodies. However, these results cannot necessarily be extrapolated to human infection, though circulating antibodies have been found in the serum of children with mycobacterial lymphadenitis[30] and in other conditions,[56] in either the presence or the absence of response to skin tests. The same caveat found in the work of Chase and Kawata applies with equal force to antigens used in serological studies.

Nevertheless, serotyping of Group II and Group III mycobacteria has elucidated better than any other means the epidemiological differences that are to be found among these strains. In a review in 1971, Runyon fully accepted this measure as a means of following organisms from environment to host[313]: in America, house dust, soil, and some animals appear to constitute the main sources of serotype VI, *M. intracellulare,* but this does not necessarily apply to human infection. Engbaek *et al.*[112] found that of 41 strains isolated from animals in Denmark, 34 were identifiable as Avian II. Of 68 British strains of various origin, over one-half belonged to Avian I or Avian II.[27] But in Japan, only 48 of 176 strains were identified as one of the avian strains, while 89 other strains fell into seven major serotypes and the remainder were very diverse.[395,396] In Czechoslovakia,[211] distributions have occurred similar to those characteristic of Britain, a considerable preponderance of Avian I or II. What is evident is that no simple statements with respect particularly to *M. intracellulare* are possible. Organisms of the Davis or VI strain appear to be widely distributed in nature but are not necessarily the ones most significant to human disease. But the distribution is not uniform among those places in which studies have been carried out, and the epidemiology of infections by any of the atypical mycobacteria is far from being complete.

4

Pathology and Pathogenesis

I. PULMONARY PATHOLOGY

Detailed and specific descriptions of gross pathology have been relatively rare. Much of the available material has consisted of resected pulmonary tissue, and post mortem examinations have most often dealt with severe disseminated disease in compromised hosts. In consequence, detailed description of the gross appearance of unmodified disease is lacking.

The problem is further compounded by the fact that pathologists have made little effort to search for features—if they exist—distinguishing among processes produced by different species of atypical mycobacteria or between any of these and tuberculosis. There is the added handicap that resected pulmonary tissue exhibits secondary alterations as a result of regimens of antimicrobial therapy. As a consequence, available material that demonstrates the natural course of these infections has been quite limited.

Race[300] pointed out very early that in the tissue he had examined (primarily pulmonary tissue and lymph nodes, predominantly infected by *M. kansasii*), histological pathology was compatible with tuberculosis but that some aspects, impossible to quantify, produced a somewhat atypical microscopic pattern. As compared with similarly resected tissue with lesions caused by *M. tuberculosis,* atypical infection seemed to produce a greater amount of fibrosis, fewer well-developed tubercles, more extensive polymorphonuclear infiltration, and less caseous and more liquefactive and fibrinoid necrosis. In addition, Race found a striking degree of nonspecific bronchitis.

In a well-devised study, Corpe and Stergus[77] sent sections of tissue from Group III mycobacteriosis to selected pathologists, together with similar material of tuberculosis. The conclusion of the panel was that it was impossible to differentiate the two conditions on the basis of the histological morphology. Subsequent reports, usually from a study of quite limited amounts of material, have confirmed the study of Corpe and Stergus.

Elston and associates,[109] for example, referred to resected tissue as presenting histological findings similar to that of ''untreated tuberculosis.'' Feldman and Auerbach[120] reported that they could discover in resected Battey-type mycobacteriosis of the lung no pattern that would permit reliable differentiation from tuberculosis. The tissues Snijder[345] examined, all but one infected by *M. kansasii,* were ''exactly like those of tuberculosis. . . . Adhesions and pleural thickening were rarely absent.'' He observed cavities, closed caseous foci, scar, and calcification, but unlike Race, he also encountered a specific, granulomatous endobronchitis. Buhler and Pollak[39] reported findings in a case caused by ''the yellow bacillus'' (presumably *M. kansasii*) in which the resected specimen revealed very dense apical adhesions. The cavity was partially lined, a finding of some interest.

In a report of the findings in 19 resected specimens of pulmonary mycobacteriosis, Merckx *et al.*[251] found cavitation in 68.4%, caseation in 84.2%, and calcification in 31.6%. The study included six infections caused by *M. kansasii,* eight by Group III mycobacteria, three by Group II mycobacteria, and two by Group IV organisms. Surrounding the lesions were nonspecific histiocytes, lymphocytes, mononuclear and plasma cells. Asteroidlike structures were observed in giant cells in five instances.

Pulmonary disease that results from some of the rarer types of mycobacterial infection—for example, *M. fortuitum* (or *M. abscessus* or *M. chelonei*)—departs widely from the lesions just described. To a certain extent, lesions are specific for the particular organisms and result from the metabolic characteristics of the agent. Specific pathology appears subsequently in the chapter devoted to each mycobacterium.

From the descriptions cited, it is evident that more precise information is necessary to a better understanding of the pathogenesis of these infections. Answers to the following questions would add greatly to the comprehension of many of the problems:

1. What is the character of the pleuritis that overlies the principal lesion? Is it granulomatous or nonspecific?

2. When pleural effusions occur, are there pleural seeding and granulomata such as occur in tuberculosis?

3. Is the dense pleuritis around the apex, as described, limited to the area of the principal lesion or is the entire pleural cavity obliterated?

4. Is the bronchitis Race observed a feature only of infection with *M. kansasii,* or does it result from or accompany other mycobacterial infections? Is it localized to the bronchi and bronchioles that drain the principal area of infection, or is it generalized (and therefore perhaps independent)?

5. Is partial lining of the cavity, as observed by Merckx *et al.,* a common feature? If it occurs with some frequency, is it possible to determine if the lining is preexistent to the infection or a part of a healing process?

6. What is the segmental distribution of lesions? Is the anterior segment of the upper lobe involved as frequently as the apicodorsal segment? When bronchogenic spread occurs, is there predilection for the superior segment of the lower lobe?

II. PATHOLOGY OF LYMPH NODES

In his early description of the pathology of lymph nodes, Race[300] was struck by a more liquefactive type of necrosis than he would have expected of tuberculosis. But the range of histological change varied from nonnecrotic, epithelioid tubercles to characteristic caseation. Jones and Campbell,[179] reporting histological observations in 15 cases of mycobacterial lymphadenitis (13 of which were caused by "chromogenic" organisms), regarded the presence of basophilic nuclear debris in the center of caseous lesions as the most characteristic feature of the infection. They also stated that edema and cellularity of the epithelioid zone and the relative paucity of giant cells produced some degree of dissimilarity from tuberculosis.

In 1969, Reid and Wolinsky[303] reviewed the reports of others and summarized their own experience. In 17 cases from which Group II (probably *M. scrofulaceum* in the majority) organisms were cultured, they observed in 4 a mixture of granuloma and suppuration, in 2 a nonspecific granulomatous reaction, and in 2 a nonspecific type of inflammation. Thus, in about half their cases, the pattern differed somewhat from that of tuberculosis, while in the other half, it was not noticeably different. In their experience, as in that of all pathologists, the range of reaction to *M. tuberculosis* is rather extensive. This study is of particular value in that it deals with a single type, if not a single species, of organism, obviously the kind of observation that becomes essential as this branch of knowledge attains maturity.

What is not established and is most difficult to learn is the rate at which disease of the lymph nodes develops. Are the differences, as reported both by individual authors and by separate authors, the result of evolution of the lesion? Is it characteristic of *M. scrofulaceum* to produce at first a fairly nonspecific inflammation, followed by granuloma, and in turn by suppuration or a mixture of suppuration and granuloma? Do infections of lymph nodes by other atypical mycobacteria follow a similar pattern but at a different rate?

III. PATHOLOGY OF OTHER TISSUES

Descriptions of the pathology produced by atypical mycobacteria in tissues other than lymph nodes or lungs are expectably rare. Weed and associates[422] found upon examination of curetted and resected osseous material only occasional tubercles. The predominant lesion consisted of nonspecific chronic inflammation, even though special staining revealed the presence of acid-fast organisms (in this case referred to as ''pigmented''). In a local case involving the distal end of the femur and extending into the knee joint, tubercles, caseation, and suppuration were all present. The changes observed did not differ from those produced by tuberculosis (at the time, the organism was identified only as a ''Group III'').[47]

Atypical nonnecrotic miliary tubercles have been encountered in the liver and the spleen. Infection by implantation—such as *M. tuberculosis* produces on the mucous membranes of the pharynx and larynx, the urinary bladder, or the bowel—seems to be very unusual if it occurs at all. Infection of most nonpulmonary and nonlymphatic structures appears as a result of extensive hematogenous dissemination in hosts with severely compromised immunity; the histological changes that result in such patients are usually much modified and frequently nonspecific.

IV. PATHOGENICITY FOR ANIMALS

All atypical mycobacteria exhibit very slight pathogenicity as measured by inoculation of the usual animals.[432] *Mycobacterium kansasii* and members of the Battey-*avium* complex usually produce no more than small, localized lesions in rabbits, guinea pigs, hamsters, rats, and mice. Strains of the Battey-avium group possess pathogenicity for chickens, depending upon the serotype,[326] and this may be enhanced by preliminary conditioning to incubation at 42°. Serial passage also enhances pathogenicity. *M. marinum* produces characteristic lesions in the tails and footpads of mice in two or three weeks. The characteristic lesions of *M. abscessus* in mice consist of abscesses of the kidney, as well as of the inner ear, with consequent "spinning disease"[19,213] Filtrates of cultures of *M. ulcerans* produce characteristic necrotic–ulcerative changes in the skin of guinea pigs.[203]

All of these observations point to a very limited pathogenicity and suggest that under ordinary conditions, atypical mycobacteria are not well adapted to the invasion of mammalian hosts. The early history of these organisms as already cited, the work of Kubica and more recent isolations from the environment (cited at length in Chapter 3), and ready isolations from the upper airways and gastric washings of humans suggest that most atypical mycobacteria are free-living organisms of the environment. Supporting the view that they are only accidentally pathogenic for man also is the great number of reactors to their antigens in comparison with the small number of humans who present evidence of disease. The striking variability of skin tests already described further argues that while colonization of the human host is relatively frequent, genuine invasion is exceptional. In these features, the problem of atypical mycobacterial pathogenicity somewhat resembles that of *Candida albicans* or strains of *Aspergillus*.

These various considerations strongly suggest that invasion of the human requires either localized or generalized impairment of mechanisms of defense. In 1949, Belcher,[22] on the basis of his experience, concluded that the aspiration of gastric and esophageal contents constituted a prerequisite to invasion of the lung by "saprophytic" mycobacteria. Gibson,[135] following a similar line of reasoning, reported a patient who had achalasia of the esophagus and who developed an acid-fast infection of the lung in close association with areas of lipid pneumonia that seemed to result from the aspiration of milk. The organism he isolated produced abscesses in the kidneys of mice but no other lesions, and Gibson concluded that the lipid material acted in a nonspecific way as an adjuvant.

Reasoning similarly that some additional condition was essential to invasion, the group at the Pasteur Institute at Lille[133] were impressed very early by the association of mycobacterial infection and pneumoconiosis. Among their first eight cases of mycobacteriosis of the lung, five patients had pneumonoconiosis. (The organisms themselves did not appear to be as important as the preexisting pulmonary damage: one was a Group I, three were Group II, and one was an avian type.) Tacquet and associates[361] subsequently demonstrated that if they subjected guinea pigs to preliminary "dusting" of the lung, either with carbon alone or with carbon containing 2% silicon dioxide, a strain of *M. kansasii* produced severe progressive disease, whereas in nondusted animals the same organisms produced either minimal or no disease. Further support for the importance of preliminary injury to the lung or impairment of pulmonary defense appeared in the retrospective study of Kamat *et al.*[183] who found among pneumoconiotic Welsh coal miners more atypical mycobacteriosis than tuberculosis.

The experiments of Barbolini *et al.*[14] involved more general mechanisms of defense. Injecting guinea pigs with cortisone 5 mg every other day, they found that two strains of atypical mycobacteria—P-1 (a strain of *M. kansasii*), and M-4 (probably *Mycobacterium marianum,* a discarded name for *M. scrofulaceum*)—produced nonnecrotic lesions in lymph nodes of injected animals, whereas without cortisone they could produce no evidence of disease in their experimental animals. In our laboratory, we observed a similar effect of cortisone in rabbits.

V. PATHOGENESIS IN HUMANS

Epidemiological aspects of mycobacterial pulmonary disease—the 3:1 ratio of males to females, the prevalence among middle-aged people, the physiological evidence offered by Ahn and associates,[3] and prevalence of the disease among miners both in Wales and in northern France—point to a strong probability that much pulmonary mycobacteriosis occurs only in individuals whose lungs have already sustained damage. Association with esophageal disease adds to the evidence that some other form of injury or injurious agents permits local invasion of an otherwise intact lung. The experimental evidence presented by Tacquet and associates adds the probability that respirable particulates, even those as nonreactive as carbon, enhance local invasiveness. The evidence thus seems sufficient to support the statement that the prerequisite to development of pulmonary mycobacteriosis is chance simultaneous occurrence both of colonies of organisms and of an impairment of local immunological mechanisms, which may be acute or chronic.

Experimental studies of more general immunological impairment have been more limited. The work of Barbolini *et al.*, however, renders it probable that the administration of cortisone during a period of colonization might well permit mycobacteria to invade. The occurrence of widely disseminated and destructive mycobacterial disease in a few subjects undergoing immunosuppressive therapy certainly establishes that the generalized impairment of immune responses permits invasion of tissue. Further experimental studies are needed to determine with precision the various kinds of immunological injury that permit the development of mycobacteriosis.

At the time of this writing, it seems a tenable view that mycobacterial disease results from a coincidence of two events: the first, a colonization by organisms in adequate numbers; the second, a localized or generalized, temporary or persistent, impairment of the mechanisms of defense.

PART II

THE PHOTOCHROMOGENIC MYCOBACTERIA

5

Mycobacterium kansasii (Hauduroy)

I. BACTERIOLOGY

This organism was first fully described as a distinct mycobacterium by Hauduroy, and it is now fully accepted as a species.[450] Bönicke's amidase tests reveal enzymes effective only against urea and nicotinamide,[33] a finding fully verified by others.[162,366] A distinctive set of lipases,[366] serotyping,[167] and phage typing[167] further establish the organism as a distinct species. For other bacteriological characteristics, see Table 2-1.

In recent years, investigators have identified nonchromogenic and scotochromogenic variants[312,366] that, except for the pigment, are identical with the photochromogenic variety. Strains with unusually weak catalase activity have also been observed.[148]

Studies of antigens of *M. kansasii* place it nearer to the tubercle bacillus than any of the other atypical mycobacteria.[226] In challenge with virulent *M. tuberculosis*, preliminary vaccination with *M. kansasii* affords greater protection than any other organisms except BCG.[278] In consequence, heterologous reactions to tuberculins and PPD are common.[286]

II. PATHOLOGY

Descriptions in Chapter 4 include the range of gross and histological observations in *M. kansasii* infections; they are not significantly different from reactions to others of the more slowly growing atypical mycobacteria.

Pathogenicity for animals is quite limited, although Hauduroy *et al.* reported a slowly progressive disease in hamsters that resulted in death in 80–100 days.[162] Most other experimental animals develop only local lesions unless some method is used to modify the animal's defensive mechanisms.

III. EPIDEMIOLOGY

A. Isolations from Environmental and Nonhuman Sources

Reference to a geographical distribution in the United States has appeared in Chapter 3. Attempts to isolate *M. kansasii* from soil and standing water have been unsuccessful.[48,206] Cultures of many samples of both raw milk and pasteurized milk and milk products have also failed to produce organisms that could unquestionably be identified as *M. kansasii*.[51,57] Tison *et al.* failed to recover the organism from the water of swimming pools but were successful in isolating it from one of 14 samples of discharge water from a hospital.[379] But from a water system in California, Bailey and associates cultured *M. kansasii* from 8 of 11 one-liter samples of tap water.[11] Froman earlier had recounted, to these investigators as well as to this writer, the fact that he had recovered low-catalase strains of *M. kansasii* from the tap water of a hospital, but the organisms of Bailey *et al.* were characteristic in all respects, including high catalase activity.

Isolations of *M. kansasii* from lower animals have been very rare. Worthington and Kleeberg[436] isolated this organism from two cows, both of which had been tuberculin-positive. One animal, at post mortem, revealed a healing granuloma of the lung, while the other had partially healing granulomas both in the lung and in the mediastinal lymph nodes. Brasher has also written[37] of the isolation of *M. kansasii* from a two-year-old heifer that had exhibited bizarre reactions to tuberculin. At autopsy, this animal showed no gross lesions, and the organism was recovered from lymph nodes that were histologically normal. Though lymph nodes of swine have most often produced isolates of the *avium*-Battey complex, Tison *et al.*[378] recorded isolation of *M. kansasii* five times from the lymph nodes of 96 swine.

B. Human Isolations

1. Geography

M. kansasii has been identified as an agent of disease in nearly all parts of the world where tuberculosis is waning and where adequate bacteriological studies have been available. Early reports of considerable numbers of patients came from Chicago,[222] Houston,[174] and Dallas.[61] Infections have also been fairly frequent in California. In Dallas, atypical mycobacteriosis of the lung has been estimated to account for as many as 14% of admissions of patients with cavitary disease of the lung and positive sputum smears.[178] In contrast, in Warring's study of pulmonary mycobacteriosis in a New England hospital,[414] atypical mycobacteriosis accounted for what seems to be less than 1% of all admissions, and of these, *M. kansasii* was the etiological agent in only one-third.

In similar contrast with the central United States, Shimoide collected only 48 cases of atypical mycobacteriosis in 14 years, of which 12% were caused by *M. kansasii*.[335] At the Brompton Hospital in London, Goldman[139] could find 25 cases of pulmonary mycobacteriosis, of which 16 were the result of infection with *M. kansasii*. Three years before Goldman's report, in Chicago, Pfuetze *et al.* had collected 152 cases of *kansasii* mycobacteriosis, and these patients had accounted for 7% of all admissions to Suburban Cook County Sanatorium.[286] At the National Jewish Hospital at Denver, by 1968, atypical mycobacteriosis was the cause of admission of 4.2% of all patients (7–8% of those with positive cultures for mycobacteria), and roughly 60% of this atypical mycobacteriosis was caused by *M. kansasii*.[123] (Since this hospital served primarily for referrals, most of the patients admitted came from adjacent states, and many of them presented specifically difficult problems in therapy.)

2. Age

With similar and somewhat overlapping data, Bates[16] reported that 63% of the armed-forces–Veterans-Administration patients were under 50 years old; Zvetina[449] reported a mean age of 48.1 years; and D'Esopo[94] described these patients as being middle-aged. From the large series of Pfuetze *et al.* in Chicago,[286] no mean age was furnished, but they were referred to as "middle-aged or elderly." Even in this series, 10.8% were under 30. The large series at Dallas[178] furnished a mean age of 48.5 years for men and 40.6 years for women; a report that represents a more widely collected series from Texas[3] provided an average age of 49 years for all patients.

3. Sex

All series so far reported demonstrate a higher prevalence among males than females. In the report of Ahn *et al.*,[3] males constituted 72%; in Goldman's[139] 84%; in that of Pfuetze *et al.*,[286] 75%; and in that of Fischer *et al.*,[123] 76%. Other series are too small, too specialized in interest, or too distorted by demographic factors (e.g., VA–armed forces) to permit conclusions. On the basis of the good agreements among the large series in which special factors were not involved, the ratio of male to female is 3:1.

In the cases of mycobacterial lymphadenitis in children, most of the reports occurred early enough so that a distinction between the types of organisms in the two sexes was not reported. In any case, the numbers with infections caused by *M. kansasii* would be too small to permit any clear distinction from other types.

4. Race

If no special factor, such as pneumoconiosis, is involved, distribution among ethnic groups appears to be proportional[54,178] to their fraction of the population.

5. Occupational and Socioeconomic Factors

Only one study, limited to Dallas County, Texas, examined this aspect of epidemiology. In that study, it was found that patients with mycobacteriosis kansasii had a significantly higher income and a measurably better standard of living than patients with tuberculosis.[54] Several patients were professional; 10 of 30 white males, at some period in their occupational history, had engaged in metal work, chiefly welding. Another 6 men had experienced some years of exposure to wood dust and paint.

The only other information pertaining to social or economic factors is inferred from the report of Lester *et al.*,[222] in which the majority of their patients were found to have suburban addresses, probably signifying better incomes and higher standards of living than those of tuberculosis patients, who cluster in the central city. Marks's report also demonstrated a prevalence higher among urban than rural people,[240] while a study in Japan places mycobacteriosis kansasii chiefly in the prefectures around the two largest cities.[336]

6. Associated Pulmonary Disease

The early report of Schepers *et al.*[328] called attention to pneumoconiosis as a possible important factor contributing to the development of pulmonary mycobacteriosis. This report, plus clinical observations at Lille,[133] led to a demonstration that the preliminary inhalation of carbon particles or of 2% SiO_2 in carbon particles produced progressive pulmonary disease in guinea pigs exposed to *M. kansasii* by inhalation. Without the preliminary "dusting" of the lung, inhalation of the organisms failed to produce disease.[361] In France,[133,362] Wales,[240] and Czechoslovakia,[269] predilection of pneumoconiotic coal-miners to infection by *M. kansasii* had been noted, although curiously enough, the infection apparently has not complicated very many cases of coal workers' pneumoconiosis in this country. In New Orleans, *M. kansasii* accounted for more than 40% of mycobacterial disease, including tuberculosis, in silicotic sand-blasters.[12]

The selectivity of mycobacterial disease for older males very early led investigators to attempt to assess the contribution of chronic obstructive pulmonary disease (COPD) to the development of mycobacterial infection. Zvetina[449] considered that there was some degree of association of the two conditions, as did D'Esopo,[94] but Bates reported COPD in only 37% of patients with infection of the lung caused by *M. kansasii*.[16] (All of these reports are derived from patients in Veterans Administration hospitals, and probably each study contains some data derived from preceding reports.) In a more representative sample of the population, including women, Christianson and Dewlett[61] encountered an incidence of 24% COPD in a group that consisted of 80% *M. kansasii* infections. Johanson and Nicholson reported an incidence of 38% previous symptomatic "other pulmonary disease" in a much larger series that represented both sexes.[178] In the largest series from Texas, Ahn *et al.*[3] found FEV_1 of less than 70% predicted in 68.9% of patients with mycobacteriosis kansasii.

There has been only slight attention to the relationship between carcinoma of the bronchus and infection with *M. kansasii*. Experience at the University of Texas Southwestern Medical School has included a rare instance in which a carcinoma, usually central, is associated with the presence of *M. kansasii* in the sputum. This finding may represent only colonization, but it may also be associated with granulomatous process. (The association, of course, is not limited to *M. kansasii* but may occur with Group II and IV mycobacteria, the avium-Battey organisms, and *M. tuberculosis*.)

IV. CLINICAL FEATURES

A. "Primary" Infection of the Lung

On the basis of analogy with tuberculosis and with mycotic diseases such as histoplasmosis and coccidioidomycosis, it might be assumed that children in contact with an adult with a sputum positive for *M. kansasii* might exhibit roentgenographic and clinical findings similar to those of primary granulomatous infections. Even if person-to-person transmission did not occur, the possibility of a common environmental source from which inhalational infection could take place would lead to the expectation of pulmonary infiltrations in children of adults with confirmed disease. Evidence that such exposure, if it occurs, results in disease in children is both meager and uncertain.

In their very extensive review of pediatric mycobacteriosis Lincoln and Gilbert encountered 13 cases of pneumonic disease, 6 associated with isolation of *M. kansasii*.[225] There were also 22 children in whom there was "any" pulmonary disease associated with any kind of atypical mycobacterium. In all of these instances, the problem was clouded by the fact that pharyngeal swabs, material aspirated through the bronchoscope, and gastric washings may present organisms that have no relation to the pneumonic process in the lung. This reservation arises from the repeated demonstration of organisms in the oral cavity and the pharynx of normal children and adults, as well as the frequency with which positive gastric washings may be obtained from healthy people.[9] Both the passage of the bronchoscope and the problems of sterilization of the instrument and its suction devices allow for the opportunity of contamination.

An example of the unreliability of pediatric secretion is the case of a 10-year-old Puerto Rican girl who reacted strongly to O.T. 1–10,000 and whose father had active tuberculosis. The roentgenogram of the child's chest revealed infiltration in the left upper lobe, associated with widening of the superior mediastinum. Cultures produced a few colonies of *M. kansasii*.[26] The circumstances were such that one would be forced to conclude that the child had a very characteristic primary tuberculosis and that the colonies of *M. kansasii* were the result of chance colonization.

On the other hand, etiology is unmistakable in the case of a newborn infant who died of massive, caseating pneumonia and whose mother also died of miliary and meningeal disease caused by "the yellow bacillus."[435] In this case, of course, the organism clearly entered the infant transplacentally. Beyond question, *M. kansasii* may be the etiological agent of pulmonary disease in children. The difficulty lies in obtaining specimens of material in such a manner as to avoid potential contamination from the upper airway and with sufficient frequency as to meet criteria for adult pulmonary mycobacteriosis, as well as to exclude other possible causes of pneumonia.

If the reverse study is undertaken—the search for evidence of pulmonary disease among children who are household contacts of patients who excrete organisms—the absence of primary pulmonary infection is striking. In over 200 children, with or without positive reactions to *kansasii* sensitin, who were in contact with sputum-positive adults, roentgenographic examination revealed no abnormal pulmonary findings. Similarly, in over 500 children who reacted to *kansasii* antigen with induration of 8 mm or more and who were less reactive, or nonreactive, to O.T. 1–1,000, no roentgenographic abnormality ascribable to mycobacterial infection could be found. One can only conclude that in spite of the high prevalence of cutaneous hypersensitivity to sensitins of atypical mycobacteria, identifiable primary inhalational infection of the lung similar to that produced by *M. tuberculosis, H. capsulatum,* or *C. immitis* is very rare.

B. Pulmonary Disease in Adults

1. Symptoms

It is the general consensus that symptoms caused by pulmonary mycobacteriosis kansasii are usually similar to, but milder than, those of pulmonary tuberculosis of corresponding extent.[222,449] In one early report, half of the patients were stated to have experienced no symptoms, and discovery of disease was the result of routine roentgenograms of the chest.[61] A later report on a much larger series reveals a similar but less marked trend toward mildness or absence of symptoms.[178] In that COPD is so common among patients with mycobacteriosis, it is evident that patients might very well fail to notice small alterations in cough, production of sputum, or malaise.

A very small proportion of patients—probably no more than 4–5%—have reported abrupt onset with high, spiking fever and severe cough. The pattern of this manifestation of disease is quite similar to that of abscess of the lung. Pleuritis, stabbing pain in the lower part of the chest, is far less common than dull, boring pain in the upper chest. Hemoptysis occurs, but figures for its frequency have limited meaning, since the amount may vary from mere streaking to free bleeding of 200–300 ml. Zvetina reported that hemoptysis occurred in about one-fourth of all patients with atypical mycobacteriosis, not distinguished by organism.[449]

Pleural effusions occur in perhaps 1–2% of patients. Fluid is usually small in amount and occurs along with extensive pulmonary disease. The "primary" effusion that has characterized tuberculosis in the past, an effusion without demonstrable disease of the lung, appears to be very rare in mycobacteriosis, if it occurs at all.

2. Physical Signs

Physical examination of the chest fails to reveal findings proportional to the disease demonstrated in roentgenograms. The location of lesions high and somewhat laterally in the lung impairs examination, while the absence of extensive exudative components tends to reduce evidence of alveolar moisture. Associated COPD, if present, may considerably over-shadow the abnormalities produced by mycobacteriosis. The most reliable finding, when present, consists of fairly marked dullness high in the chest and paucity of other expectable changes, such as rales and change in voice sounds. Compared with tuberculosis of similar extent, mycobacteriosis produces very few detectable abnormalities.

3. Laboratory Findings

Usual tests result in normal reports, except for accelerated sedimenta-tion rate. Mild leukocytosis, around 10,000, with a slight left shift, is not uncommon. In those patients who experience a pneumonic type of onset, both leukocytes and polymorphonuclears are much more numerous. Sputum stained for acid-fast organisms often reveals numerous organisms. To the microscopist familiar with *M. tuberculosis,* atypical organisms may appear sufficiently distinctive to warrant a tentative report. *Mycobacterium kansasii* is both longer and thicker; beading is heavier, even appearing at times as banding.

Skin tests may sometimes furnish a clue, according to this writer's experience, but reliable antigens are rarely available and the Communica-ble Disease Center no longer provides PPD-Y. In the opinion of others, reactions both to O.T. and to PPD are quite unreliable in differentiation[286]; at most, the results of a battery of tests with atypical antigens can be only suggestive. The diagnosis depends totally on bacteriological identification.

4. Roentgenography

While it has been maintained that mycobacteriosis is indistinguishable from tuberculosis,[335,383] and very few, if any roentgenologists would claim a high degree of accuracy in differential diagnosis from tuberculosis, sev-eral features may allow a strong suspicion of mycobacteriosis kansasii (and perhaps, to some extent, this is true of other mycobacteriosis). Most of what follows is the author's interpretation of his own experience.

1. Distal pleural disease—that is, tenting of the diaphragm and oblit-eration of the costophrenic angle—is less common than in tuberculosis,

while marked pleural reaction directly over the lesion is more striking.

2. Loss of volume of the affected segments is less apparent than in tuberculosis, possibly because of associated bullous disease and chronic bronchitis. As a consequence, upward retraction of the hilum and homolateral shift of the trachea and the mediastinum are less conspicuous.

3. Cavities occur in 85% of cases and are bilateral in 22%.[178] Characteristically, the wall of the cavity is quite thin and there is only slight pericavitary reaction.[61,286]

4. Exudative infiltrations arising from bronchogenic spreads are few and light in comparison with comparable cavitary tuberculosis. Nodulation in the segments of the lungs adjacent to cavities is usually quite sparse.[61,286]

5. In lateral films, cavities lie in front of or directly over the tracheal shadow much more often than is true of tuberculous cavities.

6. Calcifications representing healed primary infections of the lung are absent in mycobacteriosis, unless the individual has had primary tuberculosis or histoplasmosis.

No single feature alone serves to differentiate mycobacteriosis from tuberculosis, but a combination of most, or all, of these features in the roentgenogram *of a previously untreated patient* permits a strong presumption of mycobacteriosis. (The emphasis on the lack of previous treatment is essential: mycobacteriosis resembles treated tuberculosis, in that treatment tends to leave walls of cavities thin and to produce resorption of exudates.)

These remarks with respect to the roentgenogram apply only to those patients who have experienced a slow and insidious onset. Those who have abrupt and severe disease that resembles abscess or pneumonia require roentgenographic differentiation from those diseases.

Miliary and disseminated disease caused by *M. kansasii* presents the same roentgenographic problems of diagnosis as all diffuse disease of the lung. The presence of pleural effusions has particularly been noted in such cases.[146,158,246] In the more usual types of cavitary, chronic disease, Johanson and Nicholson observed a small collection of fluid in only 1 of 99 cases.[178]

When associated pneumoconiosis is present, roentgenographic features are altered, obviously. Conglomerate lesions may appear as in other complicated silicosis. Obviously, widespread nodulation of pneumoconiosis is present. Among silicotic sand-blasters, Bailey *et al.* observed greatly enlarged hilar lymph nodes in 8 of 22 patients, exudative disease occurred bilaterally in lower lobes of 5.[12]

5. Diagnosis and Differential Diagnosis

The characteristic patient is a middle-aged male of the middle class who can give no reliable history of contact with tuberculosis and whose household associates are tuberculin-negative. Symptoms will have consisted of a slight decline in weight, mild malaise and fatiguability, and perhaps a recognizable change in chronic cough or production of sputum. The physical examination will contribute little information and the roentgenogram of the chest reveals chronic cavitary disease of the lung.

Differential diagnosis must exclude tuberculosis, chronic pulmonary histoplasmosis and other mycobacterial diseases. Occurrence of disease in the central part of the United States, residence in a suburban neighborhood, and lack of travel or residence in regions of the world in which tuberculosis is prevalent or in areas in which coccidioidomycosis or histoplasmosis occurs increase the probability that the disease results from *M. kansasii*. Residence on a farm would definitely increase the chance that the etiological organism is a member of the *avium*-Battey complex[74] or possibly *H. capsulatum*.

Diagnosis depends completely upon repeated demonstration of an organism that meets the bacteriological criteria of *M. kansasii*, as well as demonstration that other potential pathogens are not present in secretions. It is most important that at least two cultures should reveal as many as 100 colonies per culture, and assurance increases with each additional culture, especially when colonies are sparse. After growth has appeared and *M. kansasii* has been verified, it is desirable to hold cultures for six to eight weeks, to allow for the possibility that *M. tuberculosis* may also be present.

Acute pneumonic forms of the disease have to be differentiated from pneumonia and from pulmonary abscess. Both in abscess and in acute mycobacteriosis of the lung, cavitation develops rather rapidly—usually in 7–10 days. But abscess occurs much more commonly in the superior segment of the lower lobe, and foul sputum does not result from mycobacteriosis.

If the roentgenogram suggests carcinoma of the bronchus, bronchoscopy and cytological study are essential, regardless of the number of positive cultures of *M. kansasii* or any other mycobacterium.

C. Disease of the Lymph Nodes

Infection by *M. kansasii* occurs most frequently in a node or a cluster of nodes that drains the oro- or nasopharynx. The most common site is the cluster at the angle of the mandible,[30] but sometimes infection occurs in the preauricular node, in which case it may be difficult to determine if the node or the parotid gland was the site of original infection.[321] Children with lymphatic disease are asymptomatic except for the appearance of the swelling, which is usually not painful. Characteristically, they are well nourished, and no antecedent history of any importance can be adduced. No contact with tuberculosis can be demonstrated and their siblings are tuberculin-negative. The great majority are between 15 and 36 months of age.

Occasional involvement of other nodes occurs. These have included—also as unilateral disease—axillary, inguinal, and postauricular clusters. In disseminated disease (see Section G below), deep nodes may be extensively involved.

The pathological changes and the course of the disease, as well as the recommended treatment, appear in Chapter 8. No evidence suggests that the lymphadenitis resulting from *M. kansasii* differs in any important respect from other atypical mycobacterial lymphadenitis.

D. Cutaneous Disease

Since *M. marinum* is photochromogenic and so specifically involves the skin, the ascription of cutaneous lesions to *M. kansasii* requires exacting bacteriological techniques. Obviously, if there is disease of deeper structures as well as of the skin, infection by *M. marinum,* which requires lower temperatures for reproduction, is almost *ipso facto* excluded.

Of the more specific processes that have been described, sporotrichoid and nodular lesions seem representative. Owens and McBride[275] reported two cases in which inoculation on the dorsum of the finger or the hand occurred. At the presumed site of inoculation, a verrucous, violaceous growth developed. Above these sites, a lymphangiitic spread occurred with resultant sporotrichoid nodulation along the forearm, but extension into the draining node did not take place in either instance. Wood *et al.* reported a very similar case of granulomatous disease of the skin.[435] Reback mentions, without description of the lesions, an infection of the skin on the hand and another on the foot that developed after two people had waded in "brackish waters" near Baltimore.[301] A nodular, granulomatous lesion of the skin, adjacent to an infected olecranon bursa, developed in an elderly man after a prick by a rose thorn.[195]

In a patient with widely disseminated infection by *M. kansasii,* including miliary lesions of the lungs, lesions resembling erythema induratum developed.[271] Macular lesions appeared on the trunk in the course of hematogenous dissemination in the patient studied by Gruhl and Reese,[152] and erythema multiforme, as well as erythema nodosum, has also been observed in hematogenous mycobacteriosis kansasii.[447] It is not indicated in any of these reports of less specific types of cutaneous response if cultures of the superficial lesions were undertaken.

E. Disease of Bone and Soft Tissue

Aside from granulomatous replacement of bone marrow in extensive hematogenous disease, *M. kansasii* has been recovered from osteomyelitic lesions of interphalangeal joints and carpal bones,[137,195] the ankle joint,[137] a vertebral body,[416] and other bones.[138,250] Lincoln's review of mycobacterial disease in children disclosed seven cases of osteomyelitis without reference to the specific mycobacterium.[225]

The development of the osseous lesion somewhat resembles that of tuberculosis in similar structures but may be more rapid. Granulomatous disease with either caseating or liquefactive necrosis is usually present and the roentgenographic alterations resemble those caused by *M. tuberculosis.* Once more, bacteriological identification of the organism represents the only reliable diagnosis.

In many instances, involvement of soft tissue represents extension from an osseous lesion, but in a patient who had received a renal homograft and intensive immunosuppressive therapy, cellulitis of the foot developed without antecedent disease of the bone. Tenosynovitis of the flexor tendons at the wrist and above it occurred in two reported cases[44,273] and in an additional patient who was seen at the VA hospital, Dallas. These were all healthy, working males. In one patient, swelling of the hand had been present for several months before the appearance of tenosynovitis.[44] In another, after the first surgical procedure, masses appeared just below and just above the elbow. In these cases, the implication is strong that some type of inoculation into subcutaneous tissue may have occurred, though a single hematogenous deposit of organisms at a site of injury cannot be completely excluded. (If these lesions indeed developed from inoculation, the course is quite different from the sporotrichoid lesions described above in Section D.)

F. Disease of the Genitourinary System

The summary by Wood *et al.* in 1956[435] included one case of bilateral disease of the kidney. The report of Fischer and others[123] included one patient whose urine repeatedly produced *M. kansasii*. In this instance, the patient manifested all the problems of severe chronic renal disease and eventually died of renal insufficiency. A very similar course is described in the report of Listwan *et al.*[230] Percutaneous biopsy of the kidney revealed chronic granulomatous disease, and a culture of this material produced *M. kansasii*. On three different occasions, biopsies yielded identical results, and the urines were consistently positive for the organism. Renal insufficiency gradually progressed to renal failure in spite of fully adequate therapy, and death resulted in the course of a year. Necropsy revealed tubular atrophy and extensive fibrosis. Since the patient had long suffered from poorly managed diabetes mellitus and since granulomatous disease was not reported from post mortem examination, it is possible that the extensive fibrosis resulted from healing of the granulomata, though the contribution of diabetes to the renal disease is not clear. Both these cases imply that the locus of the granulomas is within the renal parenchyma and that involvement of the pelvis with obstruction and pyonephrosis are less characteristic of this infection than of tuberculosis.

Because in cases of miliary tuberculosis urine may repeatedly contain the organism, the case of Phillips and Larkin[287] established that in miliary mycobacteriosis kansasii, the urine may also be repeatedly positive for the effective organism. This observation serves to emphasize the desirability of repeated cultures of the urine when one is confronted by a miliary disease of uncertain etiology.

Involvement of the epididymis and the testis was a manifestation of extensive disseminated disease in one report.[271] In the case included in the report of Merckx *et al.,* the epididymis alone was affected.[250] If extensive descending disease with granulomatous infiltration of the ureters and bladder, such as occurs in tuberculosis, results from infection by *M. kansasii,* it has not come to the writer's attention. Nor has granulomatous disease of the seminal vesicles or prostate, though disease of these structures, as well as of the ovary or the tubes, might be expected.

G. Disseminated Disease

Cases included in this category comprise those in which extensive involvement of many systems has occurred. In view of the demonstrably low virulence of the organism, it must be postulated that dissemination implies either a very large release of bacteria or some major immunological defect in the host. Review of the cases in which widespread infection has occurred confirms this impression.[115] Only one individual in the collected cases seems to have been previously healthy, although in the preceding two years he had had pneumonia, and only six months before he had had chicken-pox, a rather unusual incident in a mature young male.

In 1969, Hagmar *et al.*[158] published a review of collected cases of disseminated mycobacteriosis kansasii. Since that time, a few additional cases have appeared, but they do not change the conclusions. Among cases with *kansasii* infection, only a single pediatric patient appeared,[246] while in disseminated *avium*-Battey infection, only 2 of 11 patients were adults. Hagmar and associates further observed, as they compared the two infections, that bone marrow was less often positive for either mycobacteria or granulomas in patients with *kansasii* infections than in the other mycobacteriosis.

Hepatosplenomegaly is evident in a high percentage of patients, and some type of rash appears in about half the patients in which *M. kansasii* has become hematogenous. Generalized lympadenopathy, fairly frequent in the dissemination of organisms of the *avium*-Battey complex, has not been a feature of infection with *M. kansasii,* possibly because of differences in age. Petechiae, which might be expected, do not appear in descriptions of either disseminated disease. Anergy seems to be a fairly frequent feature of disseminated *M. kansasii,* although not all patients have been examined for this manifestation.

In peripheral blood, the outstanding feature of infection with *M. kansasii* is either pancytopenia, or anemia and leukopenia,[158] though the patient of Gruhl and Reese[152] was at first thought to have subacute leukemia. One patient had "a myeloproliferative disorder," and one had confirmed chronic granulocytic leukemia but as a result of therapy had arrived at pancytopenia.

The pediatric case is particularly illuminating in this respect: The infant was proved to have a primary lymphopenic deficiency.[246]

As mentioned before, bone marrow less frequently demonstrates organisms and granulomas than the marrow of patients with disseminated *avium*-Battey disease. However, characteristic, well-formed tuberculous granulomas should not be expected in individuals with spontaneous or iatrogenic immunological impairment. Aspirated material should receive cultural as well as microscopic study.

In view of the demonstrated lymphocytic deficiency in the pediatric case, the demonstration of anergy in many of these patients, the frequency of hepatosplenomegaly, the rather advanced age of a number of them, and the rather pervasive element of leukopenia, either spontaneous or therapeutically produced (see Table 5-1), it seems likely that the most important element in the development of this form of disseminated disease is paucity or inadequacy of thymocytes. The fact that the one patient in the collection who recovered never lost his delayed reaction[115] further emphasizes the importance of the T-lymphocyte in granulomatous disease.[49,248] That this clinical picture is not peculiar to *M. kansasii* is demonstrated in the paper of Medd and Hayhoe.[248] In association with a miliary granulomatous disease regarded as tuberculous (there was no cultural identification), they observed a similar syndrome of hepatosplenomegaly and pancytopenia in two of four patients and of a macular rash in one. Like the patients with *M. kansasii* disease, the patients in Medd and Hayhoe's group

TABLE 5-1
Disseminated Infection with *M. kansasii*

Report	Age	HSM[a]	PB[b]	BM[c]	Notes	Other
287					Miliary	
447						
Case 2	60	+	P[e]	G[h],M[i]	Anergic	Splenectomy
Case 3	61		P		Anergic	Splenectomy–cort.[j]
115	21	+	P	G,M	Pos Tbc	Recovered
271	45	+	A[f]		Miliary	Cort.; myeloprol.
230	40		P		Uremia	Diabetes
435	34				Miliary	Pregnancy
152	64	L[d]		G,M	Anergic	Leukemoid–cort.
246	5 mos					Thymic dysplasia
146	43	+	P	M	Anergic	C.G.L.–cort.
194						
Case 1	64	+			Anergic	Splenectomy–cort.
Case 2	62					
158	23		L,A[g]			

[a]Hepatosplenomegaly.
[b]Peripheral blood.
[c]Bone marrow.
[d]Liver only.
[e]Pancytopenia.
[f]Anemia.
[g]Leukopenia, anemia.
[h]Granuloma.
[i]Mycobacteria.
[j]Corticoids in therapy.

were mostly middle-aged males. In their studies, they found absolute counts of lymphocytes rarely higher than 1200. Though it may be possible that dissemination leads to suppression of the marrow, in the opinion of Kilbridge *et al.*,[194] pancytopenia in their cases certainly preceded the onset of infection.

The treatment of this form of mycobacteriosis kansasii calls for the most effective antimicrobial regimen attainable (see Section V).

Splenectomy was undertaken without effect on the course of three patients in the series, nor did corticosteroid therapy seem to affect the outcome. If the hypothesized T-lymphocyte deficiency is in fact the most significant feature of dissemination, repeated transfusions from strongly tuberculin-positive donors seems logical, although there is no report that addresses itself to this question.

V. SUSCEPTIBILITY OF *M. KANSASII* AND TREATMENT

A. *In Vitro* Tests

Strains vary in susceptibility. Investigators have not consistently employed the same methods or media, both of which are known to affect results. Table 5-2 lists antimycobacterial drugs and effective concentrations as they have been reported.

A very recent study that devotes attention to combinations of drugs as well as to single ones perhaps provides a better concept of *in vitro* effects.[384] In this investigation, the authors found that ethambutol alone is approximately the equal of isoniazid and that streptomycin is superior to either. A combination of isoniazid–streptomycin was more effective than isoniazid–ethambutol, while addition of ethambutol to isoniazid–streptomycin did not result in enhancement.

B. *In Vivo* Studies

Therapeutic trials in animals have been rare owing to the difficulty of developing a satisfactory model of disease in smaller animals. Hedgecock and Blumenthal,[164] using one strain of *M. kansasii* that was completely resistant to INH and streptomycin and a second with susceptibility *in vitro* to INH 5 μg and SM 10 μg, found that, in mice, various single and

TABLE 5-2
Susceptibility *in Vitro* of *M. kansasii*

Report	Drug	MIC[a]	Notes
427	INH	1 μg/ml	60% susceptible
	SM	10 μg/ml	83% susceptible
232	RMP	5 μg/ml	MBC[b] for 5 of 5 strains
	RMP	1.35 μg/ml	22 of 22 strains
316	EMB		
157, 261	Erythro	5 μg/ml	65% susceptible

[a]Minimum inhibitory concentration.
[b]Minimum bactericidal concentration.

combined regimens produced effects predictable from *in vitro* results, except that as a single agent streptomycin had little effect.

The experiment of Tacquet *et al.*[360] measured the effects of different agents on pulmonary disease induced in guinea pigs by preliminary "dusting," followed by inhalational infection with *M. kansasii*. Their results confirmed that isoniazid alone was ineffective but that both ethambutol and ethionamide were quite effective, ethambutol perhaps being slightly better. Isoniazid–ethambutol seemed to provide a useful combination. In a second study of the same type at the Pasteur Institute of Lille,[363] 4-4 diisoamyloxythiocarbanilid, 15 mg per week divided into six doses, markedly reduced disease.

C. Results of Clinical Treatment

Comparative clinical trials on a large scale, similar to those employed in tuberculosis, have not been attempted. Individual groups of investigators have not employed comparable doses of streptomycin (two times a week, three times a week, or daily) or isoniazid (usually 4–5 mg/kg, but sometimes 8–10 mg). Up to about 1965, the most frequent combinations consisted of isoniazid–PAS–streptomycin at varying doses, but since then ethambutol has replaced PAS, and results of all regimens are clouded by the frequent practice of surgical resection, indications for which have varied from place to place.

The few available controls consist only of patients who have refused or failed to take antimicrobial regimens. At the Brompton Hospital, of five patients who received no treatment (not all of whom had infection with *M. kansasii*), four demonstrated progression of their disease.[139] Among Dallas patients, Francis *et al.*[126] discovered four patients with mycobacteriosis kansasii who had received no drugs and whose observation had extended through 12–14 years. One of these underwent spontaneous improvement, while the other three exhibited slowly progressive disease.

Reported results of various regimens appear in Table 5-3. In some of these results, it should be noted, the end point for evaluation was six months. Certainly, some bacteriological relapses occurred after this time, and quite possibly conversion to negative may also have occurred. Longer follow-up demonstrates that after having attained satisfactory conversion of

TABLE 5-3
Conversion of Sputum, *M. kansasii*

Report	Drugs	Date[a]	Conversion
174	INH–PAS–SM	6 mos.	50%
33	INH–PAS–SM	6 mos.	50%
16	INH–PAS–SM	NS[b]	65% with surgery
123	Tailored	NS	84% (22 of 24 pts.)
178	INH–PAS–SM	NS	90%
	INH–EMB–SM	NS	

[a]Some authors used a six-month cutoff.
[b]Not stated.

sputum to negative and having maintained it for a year, about 5% of patients experience bacteriological relapses. Surgery does not alter the rate of relapse.

No protracted follow-up of the effects of regimens that included rifampin is available.

According to *in vitro* results, the best theoretical regimen one could offer for the treatment of infection with *M. kansasii* seems to be as follows:

Rifampin	600 mg daily
Ethambutol	15 mg/kg daily
Streptomycin	1.0 mg three times weekly
	(daily for severe problems)

Isoniazid at the usual dose may be added, if one desires. Even though this may seem to be the regimen most likely to produce results, it may not be significantly better than the regimen of INH–EMB–SM, for which Johanson and Nicholson recorded an 85% rate of conversion of sputum.[178]

Patients who have bacteriological relapses or who fail to convert sputum to negative by the end of six to eight months pose more difficult problems. The regimen selected depends entirely on the results of *in vitro* susceptibility. In these, as well as in very ill patients, erythromycin (250 mg q.i.d.) should be considered, and cycloserine, kanamycin or capreomycin, ethionamide, or pyrazinamide may constitute other possibilities. There seem to be no clinical trials of the carbanilid tested by Tacquet and associates.[363]

6

Mycobacterium marinum (balnei)

In 1954, Linell and Norden first isolated and identified *M. marinum* as the specific agent for a characteristic disease of the skin that was associated with swimming pools. They established the source of the infection as bacterial colonies in rough cement and described a specific response in animals as well as the histological and immunological results of human infection.[229]

I. BACTERIOLOGY

The organism is photochromogenic, grows best at 31–33°, and produces nippled colonies after 10–14 days. For further features of bacteriological identification, see Table 2-1.

Linell and Norden noted that 2 of 11 patients who had not received BCG vaccination became tuberculin-positive in consequence of their infection with *M. marinum*. Philpott *et al.*[288] likewise reported that most of their patients with *marinum* infection produced positive reactions to the rather nonspecific patch test. Of the Colorado patients originally reported, 49 were tested some years later with a battery of mycobacterial sensitins. There was a very irregular and inconstant pattern of reaction to the antigens of *M. kansasii* and *M. intracellulare* and to PPD, but 59% of the formerly infected individuals responded with reactions of 10 mm or more to the sensitin of *M. marinum*.[181] The antigenic components that resulted in cross-reactions with PPD could also be shown to produce limited but demonstrable protection against an aerobic challenge with *M. tuberculosis*.[181] It is thus evident that a suitably prepared sensitin might provide reinforcing evidence for the diagnosis but that heterologous reactions are clearly to be anticipated.

II. EPIDEMIOLOGY

All early reports dealt with infections acquired from swimming pools, either natural[263] or constructed.[229] Organisms were cultured from the water[412] or from the rough surface of the walls.[263]

Slightly more males than females acquired the disease. As might be expected, the majority of patients (86%) were between 10 and 19 years of age,[263] at least in the Colorado epidemic. Water in the pool at Glenwood Springs, the source of a great number of the American cases, was found to average 82–85°F and to be high in mineral content.[263]

Since these original observations, many sporadic infections have been observed, an interesting portion of them in association with the cleaning and maintenance of aquariums[2,15] and in one instance from a dolphin bite.[125] In the reports of aquarium-acquired infection, it had been noticed earlier that the fish were dying, although the cause was not known. Barrow and Hewitt[15] found that though cultures of water and of swabbings from the walls were unproductive, cultures from the fish themselves produced *M. marinum*.

III. PATHOLOGY

Biopsies of dermal lesions have revealed a variety of changes from frank suppuration[2,15,125,434] in sporadic cases to genuine granulomas in those associated with swimming pools.[229,263,288] Mollohan and Romer, as a result of the examination of numerous cases, reported that the earliest infiltration consisted of polymorphonuclears, which were succeeded by monocytes and lymphocytes.[263] Older lesions developed into typical tubercles, but according to Philpott *et al.*[288] and to Linell and Norden,[229] caseation did not occur. Lesions extended only as far as the corium and very rarely progressed to involve subcutaneous tissue.

Linell and Norden also described characteristic papular lesions that developed in the feet and the tails of mice two or three weeks after inoculation, and after intraperitoneal injection, Walker and associates[412] obtained such lesions, including a characteristic papular, irregular swelling they called ''bumpy tail.''

IV. CLINICAL FEATURES

The location of lesions, with few exceptions, is on the extremities. In sporadic cases derived from aquariums, the original site is often the dorsum of a finger or a hand. In the characteristic swimming pool granuloma, Mollohan and Romer reported that the elbow was the site of disease in 85% of their cases. The knee was the second most common site in this form of the disease.

Inoculation is the result of abrasion or of a puncture wound in either the epidemic or the sporadic case. Lesions appear in a variable period of from two[434] to as long as six or eight weeks,[125] but the usual time is around three or four weeks after inoculation.[263] Often, the full thickness of the skin is involved. Lesions vary from rice-grain-sized papules, usually bluish purple,[263] to suppuration and ulceration.[434] While available information is inadequate for unreserved opinion, it seems probable that the number of organisms inoculated may determine the degree of suppuration and necrosis. Certainly, the fact that the more severe and destructive processes have been associated with the presumably more heavily infected aquarium would seem to point in this direction.

A limited number of infections have been associated with ascending lymphatic extension, usually up the forearm. The distribution and appearance of the lesions produces a clinical pattern closely simulating that of sporotrichosis.

V. TREATMENT

In a study of collected reports of susceptibility of 24 strains of *M. marinum*, Van Dyke and Lake[405] provided evidence that the combined rifampin–ethambutol regimen should be the single most promising form of treatment. This treatment should be selected in all cases until the susceptibility of the individual strain is available. Except for its troublesome side effects, cycloserine would provide effective treatment, since a majority of strains are sensitive to this drug. According to Van Dyke and Lake, streptomycin and ethionamide should be effective in about 75% of infections, while one should anticipate that approximately 95% of the strains would be resistant to isoniazid.

As the discussion of susceptibility of *M. marinum* suggests, a particular strain of the organism may present an individual pattern of susceptibility. Walker *et al.*[412] obtained what they regarded as good results in seven cases with either streptomycin alone or in combination with isoniazid. After the failure of a six-week course of isoniazid, Barrow and Hewitt[15] succeeded in healing a sporotrichoid lesion by administering trimethoprim 40 mg and sulfamethoxazole 40 mg, two tablets each twice daily for one week, followed by one tablet of each three times daily for 14 days, and finally by one tablet each twice daily for 21 days. Adams *et al.*[2] secured initial improvement with a combination of isoniazid and PAS, but relapse developed after nearly eight months. After they discontinued this original regime and instituted streptomycin, healing occurred in three months. The strains Flowers[125] isolated were reported to be susceptible to cycloserine, ethionamide, and ethambutol. Wolinsky and associates[434] treated a rather troublesome sporotrichoid form of *M. marinum* infection with rifampin 600 mg and ethambutol 800 mg once daily. Improvement was evident by the end of two weeks, and complete and satisfactory healing had occurred by the end of four weeks. They continued the regime for a total of 50 days, though others[405] who recommend the same combination of rifampin and ethambutol advise continuation of therapy for 18 months or longer.

In view of these collected results rifampin–ethambutol is clearly the regime of first choice. If resistance to either of these drugs is manifest, the combination of the other one with streptomycin would seem the next preferable combination.

7

Mycobacterium simiae

In 1965, Karassova *et al.* undertook a bacteriological survey of a colony of *Macacus rhesus* in which disease was prevalent. In 33 of 69 monkeys, they found atypical mycobacteria; 42 strains originated from lymph nodes and 8 from viscera. Of these strains, 9 were originally classified as photo-chromogenic, but their enzymes were quite distinct from the other known Group I organisms, *M. kansasii* and *M. marinum,* and the colonies also differed in that they were small and dysgonic. For the new organism, they proposed speciation as *M. simiae*.[185]

I. BACTERIOLOGY

Mycobacterium simiae is niacin-positive,[185,249,445] the only atypical mycobacterium so far discovered to synthesize this substance. The small, dysgonic colonies, originally light buff, gradually turn yellow on exposure to light,[249] but the pigment is not as strong as that of *M. kansasii*.[202] Meissner and Schröder[249] seem to have encountered a few scotochromo-genic strains.

Enzymes include a vigorous catalase and an active urease but no nitrogen reductase.[202,249] Some strains hydrolyze nicotinamide and pryazinamide, but these characters are inconstant.[249] Two strains are noted to have hydrolyzed Tween.[202]

In the opinion of Schröder and Meissner, an organism isolated in

Cuba and originally declared a species as *M. habanae* is a variant of *M. simiae* and does not constitute a distinct species.

The differential diagnosis of this organism has produced some difficulty. If time for the development of pigment was not generous, color did not develop, and *M. simiae* has been repeatedly misidentified as *M. intracellulare* on the basis of enzyme activity and colonial morphology. (This emphasizes the desirability of a niacin test, even though an organism appears certain to be atypical.)

II. PATHOLOGY AND PATHOGENESIS

Of necessity, description is confined to a very limited amount of information. In the case reported by Yue and Cohen,[445] originally presented as an infection with a "niacin-positive *Mycobacterium kansasii*," the patient for a long time had received generous doses of corticosteroids for rheumatoid arthritis. He then developed progressive cavitary disease of the lungs and died. Post mortem examination revealed dense obliteration of the pleural and pericardial cavities, with numerous multilocular cavities in the lungs. Multinucleated giant cells of the Langhans type were visible in some sections, but there were no tuberculoid granulomas in the walls of the cavities, and the greater part of the inflammatory reaction consisted of "an unusual epithelioid cell response."

In the instance of a second patient,[99] histological examination of pulmonary tissue resulted in more characteristic tuberculoid granulomas and caseation. The anomalous histological findings in the first case, therefore, seem more likely to result from effects of corticosteroids than from some characteristics of the organism.

Experimental studies in small animals appear not to have been undertaken. The monkeys of the original study apparently presented characteristic tuberculosis. Similar monkeys in their native habitat have twice demonstrated infection with this disease.[425]

III. EPIDEMIOLOGY

There is relatively little epidemiological information. In the report of Donovan and associates,[99] the patient had handled monkeys and their tissues for a number of years, but they also reported isolations of *M. simiae* from seven other persons. It seems entirely possible that infected *Macacus* might transmit this mycobacterium to man.

IV. CLINICAL FEATURES

In the patient of Yue and Cohen, infection with *M. simiae* pursued a course marked by rapid progression and extensive pulmonary cavitation. Almost certainly the disease was exacerbated by the corticosteroids he had received. The patient of Donovan *et al.* was found to have atelectasis and infection of the lingular segment as a feature of carcinoma of the bronchus. The patient of Krasnow and Gross,[202] an 88-year-old female, suffered extensive bilateral disease with numerous cavities and extensive fibrosis and infiltration. Since cultures of her sputum also at times produced *M. fortuitum*, the individual contribution of each organism is impossible to assess with any accuracy.

V. SUSCEPTIBILITY AND THERAPY

Strains of *M. simiae* are resistant to all the usual drugs.[202] Choice of antimycobacterial agents would consequently involve the same problems as occur in the management of strains of the *avium*-Battey complex. Tests *in vitro* should include pyrazinamide, cycloserine, capreomycin, and kanamycin, as well as tetracyclines and erythromycin.

PART III

THE SCOTOCHROMOGENIC MYCOBACTERIA

8

Mycobacterium scrofulaceum

Recognition of pigmented acid-fast organisms dates to the end of the last century. Although they had been found in human secretions, Pinner demonstrated that these organisms also might be recovered from taps and from scrapings from faucets. In his opinion, they were similar in bacteriological properties to mycobacteria isolated from dermal lesions of cows (see Chapter 1).

In 1956, Weed *et al.* identified a pigmented mycobacterium[423] as the etiological agent of a form of lymphadenitis in children, and in the same year, Prissick and Masson collected a number of instances of this disease, identified the organism as a member of Runyon's Group II, and proposed the name *M. scrofulaceum.*[296]

I. BACTERIOLOGY

On the usual media, *M. scrofulaceum* appears in the form of compact, domed colonies of a strong yellow-orange color, which gradually deepens as exposure to light occurs. Flecks of red carotenoid pigment appear against the yellower background. Growth is usually complete by 10–14 days. In liquid media, organisms are randomly oriented and present no semblance of cording. Other similar pigmented organisms may form either domed and rounded colonies or a spreading, butyrous growth.

In stained preparation, organisms of Group II appear longer, thicker, and more coarsely beaded than *M. tuberculosis*.

If scotochromogenicity is an established feature of the bacterium under study, the first step calls for the differentiation of *M. scrofulaceum* from other species and strains of the group. Wayne *et al.* found that hydrolysis of Tween 80 represented a simple and practical means of separating environmental mycobacteria (hydrolyzers) from pathogenic types (nonhydrolyzers).[421] Kubica and the leading American authorities regard this test as a valid and satisfactory one.[205,207] A Japanese study group has added a rather simple additional confirmatory test in the form of susceptibility to ethambutol.[452] Susceptibility characterizes the tap-water organisms and other environmental scotochromogens, while *M. scrofulaceum* is resistant.

Various other features assist in differentiation. The amide series of Bönicke[33] establishes *M. scrofulaceum* as a weak hydrolyzer of urea, and its catalases[6] and phosphatases[5] differ somewhat from those of other organisms. Lipid analysis[176] leads to a series of patterns among Group II organisms. This mode of study establishes relationships between the *avium–intracellulare* complex, *M. xenopi,* and *M. scrofulaceum,* all of which have similar patterns. *Mycobacterium aquae,* though not universally accepted as a species, has a distinct pattern, as does *M. gordonae.* There is also a specific pattern assigned to *M. flavescens.*

The results of this type of study underscore the problems of classification and identification. It is evident, for example, that in lipid composition the organism of scrofula may be structurally and bacteriologically closer to the *avium*-Battey complex than to other scotochromogens, and there are other strains or species that occupy an area still closer to the Group III pathogens. Serotyping of Group II organisms, at least for the present, seems to offer the most useful solution. Bel,[21] in a comparison of serotyping with Adansonian classification, found that 41 of 51 strains of scotochromogens isolated from human lymph nodes serotyped as *M. scrofulaceum,* while 4 each serotyped as strains Lunning or Gause. These 2 latter strains by Adansonian analysis are regarded as varieties of *M. aquae nonurealyticum* (apparently in Bel's nomenclature the same as *M. gordonae*). Obviously, these procedures are available only in laboratories devoted to research in mycobacteriology. For others, it is recommended that the steps outlined in Table 2-2 be followed in the classification of Group II mycobacteria.

II. PATHOLOGY AND PATHOGENESIS

Descriptions of abnormal changes in lymph nodes affected by atypical mycobacteria have not undertaken the fine points of differentiation, if any exist, among Runyon's groups. If the lesions produced by *M. scrofulaceum* differ importantly from the lesions caused by other atypical mycobacteria, there is no available information. Indeed, pathologists have for the most part maintained that there is little, if any, difference between lesions caused by atypical organisms and those caused by *M. tuberculosis*.

Reporting studies of a group of lymph nodes predominantly infected by *M. kansasii* but including both scotochromogenic and nonchromogenic strains, Race[300] felt that polymorphonuclear leukocytic infiltration was more prominent and edema more striking than he usually encountered in tuberculosis in lymph nodes. Jones and Campbell[179] studied the pathology of lymph nodes that were principally the result of "nonchromogenic" mycobacterial infection and found two or three points of interest: an unusual amount of basophilic nuclear debris in the center of necrotic areas; an unusual edema and cellularity of the reaction; and a relative paucity of giant cells. In the report of Merckx *et al.*,[251] mycobacteria of Group II were stated to have produced liquefactive rather than caseous necrosis.

The portal of entry in children with mycobacteriosis of the cervical nodes appears from anatomical considerations to be some site in or about the oropharynx, perhaps including the middle ear. It has already been shown that repeated isolations of atypical mycobacteria have resulted from cultures of material from the oropharynx. In East Anglia,[355] Australia,[337] and Texas,[157] cultures have established the presence of strains of atypical mycobacteria in throat swabs or tonsils of healthy children. In the Texas study, one child whose submandibular node produced a heavy growth of *M. kansasii* also underwent tonsillectomy and adenoidectomy. Both tissues, though they showed no histological evidence of granuloma, contained *M. kansasii*.

Since none of the children in the Texas study presented any abnormality of the lungs, it appears that the "primary" infection was in fact in the upper rather than the lower airway.

If one compares the number of isolations from healthy individuals at any one time with the incidence of clinical mycobacterial scrofula, it becomes evident that only a relatively few children develop manifest disease.

It would be logical to suppose that some additional factor enters into the circumstances that permit invasion. In some of these reports, though by no means all of them, it seems as if some bacterial or viral pharyngitis may have preceded the onset of mycobacterial disease in the nodes. The distribution by age, mostly between one and three years, coincides with a period of striking oral exploration of the environment, and opportunities of infection would presumably be high. It may also correspond with a period of frequent immunizations, with possible immunological preemption.

III. EPIDEMIOLOGY

A. Environment

Early reports did not undertake to distinguish *M. scrofulaceum* from other scotochromogenic mycobacteria. The report of Kubica *et al.*[206] of cultures of soil and water in Georgia revealed that samples contained numerous Group II as well as Group III mycobacteria, and similar results developed from cultures in Texas, though the number of samples was much smaller. In Turkey, similar samples of soil and water taken from around Ankara produced many strains, of which 16% were classified as Group II.[156] Much more recent studies of similar material in Japan have led to the identification of three different types of Group II organisms; the most numerous strains meet the criteria for *M. aquae*.[403] Isolations of various strains from tap water have occurred from the first environmental studies and continue to be frequent down to the present.[11]

Other sources of infection or colonization have received less attention. Cultures of raw milk from refrigerated tanker trucks produced 49.9% positive cultures for mycobacteria in winter samples, twice the rate of isolation in the spring samples, and three times that of summer samples.[51]

In the cultures of aliquots obtained during the winter, 84% of all scotochromogenic strains were found, and most of the 95 strains isolated from winter samples failed to hydrolyze Tween 80. In France, a study of the sediment of raw milk likewise produced many positive cultures, of which a considerable number proved to be scotochromogenic.[369]

B. Secretions and Tissues of Healthy Humans

This subject has already received notice in the discussion of pathogenesis and in the chapter on early history. In the Australian study, 30 positive cultures from 441 pairs of removed tonsils resulted in 17 strains of Group II, 9 strains of Battey organisms, and four Group IV types.[337] Stewart *et al.*[355] obtained only 10 isolations from 789 pairs of tonsils; of these, 6 were identified as *M. xenopi,* 2 as Group II, and 2 as *avium-*Battey. However, all isolations were derived from 246 pairs of tonsils removed during March, April, and May. The variation in proportions of organisms between Australia and England is striking.

Among patients in Japanese sanatoriums, Yamamoto and associates repeatedly recovered Group II mycobacteria from the sputums of 153 of 188 people who excreted any type of atypical mycobacteria.[442] These isolations, however, apparently reflected colonization of previously damaged lungs. When the Japanese investigators applied their criteria for mycobacterial disease of the lung, only 51 patients remained, and of these, 49 excreted *M. intracellulare.*[396,452] The import of the study is only that scotochromogenic mycobacteria are frequent contaminants of the oropharynx or airways of people resident in Japan.

C. Human Reactions to Sensitins

Soon after the production of PPD-B, a sensitin for Group II was developed and designated as PPD-G (Gause strain). In 1957, Edwards and Krohn[105] reported results of tests with this and other mycobacterial sensitins in India and the Philippines. Results varied considerably with respect both to age and to place, and the investigators failed to identify a region in which scotochromogenic sensitization appeared to play a dominant role in nonspecific sensitization.

Later, in Norway, Bjerkedal[29] carried out a study with 10 mycobacterial sensitins. Among schoolchildren, he found 14.1% reacted to PPD-G, but responses varied widely from place to place, and it was difficult to determine by this method what might be the most prevalent sensitizing mycobacterium. In general, wherever sensitization to PPD-G was slight, reactions to other sensitins were also weak.

In a similar trial of a battery of sensitins in South India, Wijsmuller and associates[429] noted that the prevalence of sensitization as measured by PPD-G increased as the age of the child increased and that both very small and very large reactions characterized male as opposed to female children. In much the same vein as Bjerkedal, these authors concluded that ''low grade sensitization to tuberculin is caused by a group of nontuberculous mycobacteria rather than by a single species'' but that all these atypical mycobacteria in antigenic composition resembled the Gause strain rather than *M. tuberculosis*.

The report of Runyon and Dietz[315] explains in part the inadequacy of skin tests as an epidemiological tool for study of the epidemiology of scotochromogenic sensitization. They injected guinea pigs with a strain of scotochromogenic mycobacteria and tested with multiple antigens. Of the animals injected, 4 reacted more strongly to avian than to the homologous sensitin, while 10 responded too poorly to any antigen to permit discrimination. Of the remaining 39 guinea pigs, 24 reacted predominantly to the sensitin of *M. scrofulaceum* and 15 to that of *M. aquae*.

D. Distribution of Human Disease

1. Geography

From the preceding discussion, it is evident that the distribution of *M. scrofulaceum* and its principal manifestation, lymphadenitis in children (Table 8-1), vary widely from place to place and that in a number of places it is not the predominant cause of mycobacterial scrofula. In the Great Lakes region, Canada, and Japan, *M. scrofulaceum* appears to be the predominant pathogen for lymphadenitis, but this is not true of England and Wales.

TABLE 8-1
Lymphadenitis in Children: Mycobacteria Involved by Location

Report	Place	scrofulaceum	intracellulare	avium	photo	tuberculosis
179	Melbourne, Austr.	13			2	
45	Western Australia	3	12			
296	Canada	100%				
250	Rochester, Minn.		Mixed			
69	St. Paul, Minn.	100%				
431	Cleveland, Ohio	8	1			
90	Columbus, Ga.	6	2			
1	Oklahoma	3	?			
30	Dallas, Texas	3	2			
326	Wales		12		8	
319	Japan	4		4		
358	Africa					100%[a]

[a]Undoubtedly *M. tuberculosis* produced lymphadenitis in other areas than Africa, but reports dealt primarily with the disease resulting from atypical mycobacteria, and hence reliable comparison is difficult.

Around the Melbourne region, *M. scrofulaceum* produces most of the infections, but not in Western Australia.

2. Age, Sex, Race, and Family

Without regard to the specific organisms, most cases of mycobacterial lymphadenitis occur between the ages of one and three years, with only a scattering—frequently involving other than cervical nodes—in older children. Lincoln and Gilbert's[225] extensive summary of 477 cases (as of 1972) indicates that sex and race play little role in epidemiology. In only 5 instances was more than one child affected in the same family.

3. Associated Disease

The review cited[225] and experience in Texas do not permit any conclusions with respect to provocative or adjuvant factors that might lead a specific child to develop disease. Some of the possible contributing conditions have received attention in discussion of the portal of entry. To these one might add the consumption of increasing quantities of milk and water, if these are the substances through which colonization is established. Every report seems to indicate that children who develop mycobacterial scrofula have not exhibited undue susceptibility to other infections and have generally been healthy. In only four instances did the cited review find reports of abnormal films of the chest, and there is no assurance that the same organism affected the lung as involved the cervical node.

IV. CLINICAL FEATURES

A. Lymph Nodes

Mycobacterial lymphadenitis is usually confined to a cluster of nodes or to a single node in the submandibular area. Other nodes frequently involved include the preauricular and occasionally those of the posterior cervical triangle.[321,407] In the review of Lincoln and Gilbert, among 477 cases of lymphadenitis, in 9 instances axillary nodes were affected, in 12 inguinal nodes, and in 3 cases, epitrochlears. In only one patient was there bilateral involvement.

Enlargement of the affected node develops rather gradually, usually extending over three or four weeks. There is no important effect on general health and pain seems to be slight. If treatment is delayed, the infection eventually points to the surface, perforates, and forms a draining sinus. Eventually, if no intervention takes place, calcification may occur.[1,30]

Differential diagnosis must exclude infection by *M. tuberculosis*. The normal roentgenogram of the chest,[358] involvement of a single node or a cluster on one side, lack of exposure to known tuberculosis (easily traceable in the young child), negative tuberculin reactors among siblings,[30] a frequently superior socioeconomic position,[54] and reaction to mycobacterial sensitins larger than PDD[1,406] should cause one to consider the most likely agent to be one of the atypical mycobacteria. For comparative purposes, it is instructive to compare the findings of Sula and associates in Africa.[358] They found *M. tuberculosis* in 41 isolates from 57 cervical nodes, and no atypical mycobacteriosis. Half of the affected children were 10 years of age or older.

Boyd and Craig[36] have raised the question of the relationship between atypical mycobacteriosis of the lymph nodes and cat-scratch disease. The histological appearance is much the same, and probably only a demonstration of organisms in sections of tissue would permit differentiation,[303] though employment of cat-scratch antigen might provide diagnostic information. However, these authors were able to isolate "photochromogens" in seven of their eight patients and "scotochromogens" from the eighth. Obviously, the question is not fully resolved, though it should be relatively easy to determine if both diseases are the result of the same organisms.

The treatment of mycobacterial lymphadenitis is clean and complete excision of the node or the cluster of nodes, together with the overlying skin if a sinus has formed.[321] The use of drugs in association with surgery has been widely practiced,[55,90,321,406] but Wolinsky presented evidence to suggest that antimicrobial therapy is unnecessary,[433] and Abello and others did not employ drugs with any consistency.[1] In eight infections treated, they encountered a single recurrence four years later. In a large series from Dallas, 38 patients were treated with antimicrobials and surgery with no relapses.[321] In fact, however, none of these series is really comparable. At Cleveland, nearly all the infections were caused by *M. scrofulaceum,* while in the Texas cases, the agent was predominantly *M. kansasii*. The use of antimicrobials, therefore, will have to remain *sub judice*.

B. Lung and Pleura

What appears to represent primary infection of the lung has been reported three times to have occurred in young children. In the first of these cases, there was no apparent lymphadenopathy, the process being limited to the lung and associated with obstructing endobronchitis. Bronchoscopy revealed striking granulomatous stenosis, and aspirated material contained a Group II organism. Though the mycobacterium was identified as *M. scrofulaceum,* its antibiotic susceptibility was very unusual for that species.

Three cases—one in a child of six years,[88] a second in a child of five years, and the third in a 10-month old infant[204]—in many respects resembled a postprimary dissemination following inhalational infection. In the older of these, though disease was widely disseminated, roentgenograms of the chest revealed scattered, patchy pneumonic infiltrations. The youngest patient was found to have a segmental pneumonia associated with increased hilar densities. Resemblance to some of the patterns observed in "primary" tuberculosis was evident.

Among adults, pulmonary disease in association with Group II organisms is very difficult to assess. In clinics for tuberculosis, it is by no means rare to discover mycobacteria in the sputum of a patient who had been negative for several years as a result of successful treatment of tuberculosis. These prove to be pigmented mycobacteria, in most instances *M. gordonae.* However, the appearance of organisms in the sputum is not associated with roentgenographic changes or with any evidence of illness. In many cases, the infection or colonization lasts for months or years without any apparent effect on health. So far as can be determined, the appearance of these organisms in the sputum does not require intervention.

On the other hand, some of these infections are undoubedtly serious.[433] Gernez-Rieux and Tacquet's report exemplifies this type of infection.[133] Scotochromogenic organisms were found in the sputum of three of five pneumoconiotic miners and evidently produced alterations both in health and in the roentgenograms. It seems beyond question that in the presence of some particulates, such as silicon dioxide, the danger of infection is greatly enhanced. Apparently, the infection in the presence of SiO_2 may prove lethal, as reported in a conference at Brighton, Utah. In that instance, a silicotic miner, having developed pulmonary disease caused by Group II organisms, succumbed to a miliary dissemination.

A somewhat doubtful instance of infection of the pleura by Group II organisms was reported by Bhadrakom *et al.*[25] The patient was an adult male who was very ill with what was thought to be cirrhosis of the liver, possibly associated with hepatoma. One of several pleural aspirates produced a culture of scotochromogenic organisms. No other similar primary pleural infection has been reported.

C. Cutaneous Lesions

Aside from lesions of the skin in association with chronically draining deeper tissues, such as bone or lymph node, infection of the skin appears to be quite rare. Only one instance has reached notice, that of a young male, whose lesion consisted of a small papule located on the elbow. Histological examination revealed neither tubercle nor necrosis, but culture resulted in the growth of a scotochromogenic mycobacterium, not otherwise identified.[197]

D. Bone and Soft Tissue

Most of the reports deal with osteomyelitis in multiple sites, usually with some other evidence of disseminated disease, and they are discussed under that heading. The literature contains accounts of a few localized infections, however.

An Australian report describes the onset of redness and swelling around an ankle four months after the injection of cortisone for an original complaint of pain. Histological examination revealed poorly formed tubercles, and cultures resulted in the isolation of a Group II organism.[68] There was apparently no osseous destruction.

Three of the patients reported by Kelly *et al.*[190] appeared to have infection of bone or soft tissue caused by scotochromogenic mycobacteria.

In one of these, infection developed after laminectomy and resulted in abscess and partial destruction of the bone around the lumbosacral joint. The others were found to have granulomatous disease involving, the deltoid bursa in one and in the other, the prepatellar bursa.

E. Disseminated Disease

Weed and associates reported the case of a 16-year-old boy who developed numerous draining sinuses from a low-grade osteomyelitis that affected frontal and parietal bones, a scapula, an ulna, a tibia, 10 ribs, and several metacarpals. Group II organisms were recovered at various times from all of these sites. The histological features consisted chiefly of chronic inflammation and fibrosis, with only slight granulomatous changes.[424] A somewhat similar case in a six-year-old girl was described by Yamamoto et al.[442] Widely disseminated involvement of bone also occurred in the case reported by Danigelis and Long[88] and in one case of Krieger et al.[204] One of the patients in the latter report formed nonnecrotic tubercles that histologically resembled sarcoidosis, and the diagnosis was made only after organisms were cultured. The second case reported by Krieger and his associates involved a 10-month-old child who exhibited generalized lymphadenopathy, together with pain, redness, and swelling around one ankle joint. The periosteum was elevated but there appeared to be little or no reaction in the bone. Drainage resulted in the isolation of a scotochromogenic mycobacterium. All of these infections subsided, in the case of Weed et al. as a result only of drainage and debridement, without assistance of drugs. One of the others was treated with drainage and INH–PAS, while the other two received INH–PAS–SM.

Disseminated disease without involvement of the bone has also occurred. (Because of problems of identification of organisms, there is no certainty which of these several cases had infection with M. scrofulaceum and which with other mycobacteria of Group II. When the infecting agent has been more fully identified, that fact is noted.) In the first of these,[180] a young child with thrombocytopenia of unknown origin received 15 mg of prednisone daily. A scotochromogenic organism was subsequently cultured from the bone marrow and, as the disease progressed, from drainage from the middle ear, from the urine, and again from marrow. The liver and the spleen eventually became greatly enlarged and the pathological picture closely resembled Letterer–Siwe disease. In the other instance, a hydrocephalic child received various shunting catheters and eventually developed meningitis as a consequence of infection with an organism identified as *M. aquae*. The organism was also recovered from cultures of ascitic fluid. In this and in some of the other instances described in this section and in Section IV.D. one cannot overlook the possibility that the organism may have been introduced from without.

Disseminated disease in adults is almost invariably associated with some other serious disease. Relationship to silicosis has already received notice. One of the two cases reported by McCusker and Green[247] apparently had chronic granulocytic leukemia, for which he received myeleran. In the course of therapy, he developed miliary disease of the lungs and died. Examination post mortem revealed miliary disease with poorly organized epithelioid granulomas affecting all viscera. Similarly, the case reported by Zamorano and Tompsett occurred in a patient with pancytopenia who died very rapidly of a disseminated infection.[447] Autopsy revealed miliary disease throughout the viscera, with very large and necrotic mediastinal lymph nodes as a particularly striking feature. From all sites, a scotochromogenic mycobacterium was recovered. While not providing a full report, Kuo and Roshi examined a spleen removed at surgery, in which miliary tubercles were present.[212]

Quite remarkable is the unusual prevalence in Japan of meningitis. Yamamoto and colleagues[442] encountered five cases of meningitis, and in one of these, miliary disease was also present.

V. SUSCEPTIBILITY AND TREATMENT

A. Tests *in Vitro*

It has already been noticed that classification of organisms in Group II is as yet uncertain or incomplete and that until better identification is obtainable, studies and reports may well include observations on two or more species. The fact that only recently has *M. szulgai* been recognized as a species increases further the likelihood that some of the accounts described above as well as some of the statements with respect to susceptibility may have included this organism.

Studies of the susceptibility of Group II organisms have been somewhat less numerous than those of strains of Group I or Group III, primarily because the infections are much less common. However, in 1961, Virtanen reported that about two-thirds of 38 strains of scotochromogens were sensitive to PAS and about half of them were also susceptible to kanamycin and to sulfadiazine.[409] Guy and Chapman also reported that some Group II strains were inhibited by 5 mg/ml erythromycin but not by tetracyclines or chloramphenicol.[157] An extensive study of many strains by Hobby et al.[167] revealed that strains of Group II mycobacteria were variously susceptible to the more commonly employed antituberculosis agents: INH, PAS, SM, and sometimes cycloserine or ethionamide. Tsukamura also reported that tap-water scotochromogens were susceptible to ethambutol, though M. scrofulaceum was not. Hawkins and McClean[163] reported that many strains of scotochromogenic organisms were susceptible to a range of concentrations of cycloserine.

B. Effects in Human Disease

Since there are no trials in animals that would add measurably to choice of antimycobacterial agents, trials in humans furnish the best evidence of efforts. Since most cases of colonization of the lung receive no treatment and since Wolinsky made it evident that scrofulous nodes, properly managed surgically, probably require no antimicrobial therapy, the test cases consist of patients with disseminated disease.

In the case reported by Gonzales et al.,[140] in which meningeal and peritoneal infection were associated with a shunt for hydrocephalus, a change in catheters may have been the effective measure. However, the child also received continuous therapy, at first with SM–PAS–INH and later with INH–EMB.

The case reported by Danigelis and Long,[88] who presented multiple infection of the long bones as well as of the small bones of the feet and hands, received INH–PAS–SM as original treatment. Marked improvement was observed. After 18 months, SM and PAS were discontinued and he received INH alone. Relapse occurred.

In the case of a 3-year-old child with thrombocytopenia of unknown cause, Joos *et al.*[180] undertook to treat the organism, identified as the "Gause" strain, with kanamycin and ethionamide. These produced no benefit. A 10-month-old child with generalized lymphadenopathy and a single site of osteomyelitis apparently recovered as a result of a regimen of INH–PAS.[204] A case of what appeared to be primary pulmonary disease caused by *M. scrofulaceum* failed to improve during a two-month treatment with INH–PAS, but improvement became manifest after the initiation of a regimen that included rifampin, ethambutol, ethionamide, and isoniazid. Improvement, however, was very gradual, and it might have been the result of natural defenses rather than of the regimen.

Adults with disseminated disease usually have had other very severe diseases, sufficient in themselves to result in death. It is impossible to form any conclusions from the antimicrobial regimens they received.

On the basis of the collective experience, plus the information available from studies *in vitro,* it would seem reasonable to initiate treatment in severe and threatening disease with a combination of INH–SM–CS and rifampin, until reports of the susceptibility of the individual strain become available. If the strain seems to be *M. gordonae,* ethambutol should be included and cycloserine omitted.

9

Mycobacterium szulgai

Mycobacterium szulgai, which closely resembles *M. gordonae,* was identified as a pathogen by Marks *et al.* in 1972.[242]

I. BACTERIOLOGY

When *M. szulgai* is cultured at 25° it exhibits photochromogenicity, but it is entirely scotochromogenic at 37°. On standing, as is true of other pigment-forming organisms, the color gradually deepens, and flecks of red—carotenoid pigment—appear. It differs from *M. gordonae* in the patterns of its lipids, and serologically it is distinct from other mycobacteria. The organism has been found to hydrolyze Tween and to possess arylsulfatase, nitrate reductase, and a strong catalase[242] (see Table 2-2).

II. PATHOLOGY

The pathological lesions produced by *M. szulgai* apparently do not differ in any important way from the lesions that result from other atypical mycobacteria.

III. EPIDEMIOLOGY

Recognition and description of the organism are so recent that little information is available. Evidently, its distribution is widespread, since infections have occurred in Japan and Wales and in Cleveland, Ohio. It is very possible that a number of infections with scotochromogenic organisms reported in the past may have involved *M. szulgai*.

IV. CLINICAL FEATURES

All American cases so far identified have had pulmonary disease with the usual range of relatively mild to moderate constitutional complaints and pulmonary symptoms.[327]

Among the seven cases reported by Marks *et al.*,[242] four were pulmonary, one involved cervical lymph nodes, and two were infections of the olecranon bursa.

V. SUSCEPTIBILITY AND TREATMENT

Available strains revealed variable sensitivity to isoniazid 1 $\mu g/ml$, but nine strains were susceptible to streptomycin 10 $\mu g/ml$. The same nine strains also were susceptible to the following drugs at the concentrations indicated:

RMP, 5 μg
EMB, 10 μg
ETH, 5 μg
VM, 5 μg—slight resistance
CM, 10 μg—slight resistance

The five American patients with pulmonary disease all responded satisfactorily to varying regimens. Three received rifampin in some combination; one received a brief regimen of SM–PAS–INH, although he had earlier been treated with these same drugs; the fifth patient received INH–

PAS. All achieved negative cultures.[327] On the basis of these few reports, rifampin should be included in every regimen, unless tests indicate outright resistance. To it one might add streptomycin and either ethambutol or isoniazid, as studies *in vitro* would indicate.

PART IV

THE NONPHOTOCHROMOGENIC MYCOBACTERIA

10

The *Avium*-Battey Complex

In 1967[313] and again in 1971,[314] Runyon stated succinctly the problem that mycobacteriologists have almost unanimously recognized: "*M. intracellulare* and *M. avium* so much intergrade that reference is better made to the avium complex." In spite of this statement, it is generally accepted that *M. intracellulare* is a species, and it is so described. However, it is a species with a very broad range of characters. At one end of the range resemblance to *M. avium* is striking, at the other it seems to merge with organisms of the soil that possess no pathogenicity.

I. BACTERIOLOGY

Specific identifying characteristics of the principal members of the complex have been set out in Table 2-3. Organisms of Group III vary widely in pathogenicity, and the first step in identification calls for separation of those species that rarely produce disease (*M. terrae, M. gastri,* and *M. triviale*) from the more pathogenic members of the complex. Selkon,[333] in agreement with several others,[205,207] decided upon hydrolysis of Tween as a reliable criterion: organisms that possess the hydrolase are nonpathogenic. This test may be supplemented by the tellurite reduction test, which is positive in the case of the pathogenic organisms and negative in those that hydrolyze Tween.[207]

By chemical means, Smith and others[341,342] attempted to identify lipids of such specificity as to serve as species markers, but these compounds of Group III organisms proved to be too heterogeneous to permit classification. In Tsukamura's extensive battery of biochemical tests, the mycobacteria of this complex again proved refractory to systematization, though results were somewhat better.[388]

The method of serotyping by agglutination and agglutinin absorption developed by Schaefer[324] has seemed to provide a better working order than the several other methods. On the basis of present evidence, the complex consists of two types of avian organisms and a considerable number of other strains that are distinguishable by serotyping. Runyon[314] stated that in the United States serotype VI appears in house dust, soil, lower animals, and surface waters. A similar organism has been encountered in similar distribution in Czechoslovakia,[187] but the investigations of Kubin and colleagues[211] established further that the organism once identified as the species "*M. brunense*" is in fact identical with serotype "Davis," also widely distributed in the environment in Czechoslovakia. In a study of 68 strains of Group III organisms, serotype was compared with a variety of other characters, including biochemical and enzymatic traits, lipids, and susceptibility to drugs. Classification as derived from these other features did not correspond well with established serotypes.[27]

Neither the temperatures at which serotypes grow best nor pathogenicity for birds serves adequately to distinguish strains. One strain isolated from human tissue, *M. avium* "Chester," preferentially grows at 45° and serotypes as an avian strain, but it is not pathogenic for birds. On the other hand the strains isolated and studied by Kubin *et al.*,[209] which serotyped as Avian II, had bacteriological characteristics like those of *M. intracellulare*, grew best at 37°, but were pathogenic for chickens and rabbits.

For the present, serotyping seems to be the most acceptable method for characterization of Group III organisms. But it appears that members of the complex are relatively undifferentiated and possess extraordinary plasticity in the face of varying environments and hosts, which have included, soil, water, birds, and mammals. The decision to employ the term *complex* seems fully justified. From the clinical viewpoint, no further characterization is necessary, though as serotyping becomes more widely used, it may become possible to distinguish the specific features of disease or of epidemiology of particular strains.

II. PATHOLOGY AND PATHOGENESIS

According to Corpe[74] and to numerous other reporters,[183,344] gross pathology produced in humans by *M. intracellulare* does not differ in any important fashion from that produced by *M. tuberculosis*. Corpe and Stergus, in order to obtain unbiased study of histological features of the disease, sent sections from resected pulmonary tissue to 27 consultant pathologists, none of whom were able to perceive any identifying characteristics.[77] Smyth *et al.*,[344] Feldman and Auerbach,[120] and Selkon have all concurred, but Engbaek and associates noted an extensive and unusual infiltration of the bronchial submucosa by many lymphocytes and plasma cells, although the pulmonary lesions themselves resemble tuberculosis.[111] Lesions in the lymph nodes of pigs are described as "indistinguishable from tuberculosis."[373]

With respect to the infection as it occurs in human lymph nodes, Reid and Wolinsky[303] found that lesions of the *avium*-Battey complex could not be distinguished from those of *M. tuberculosis,* bearing in mind that the human organism produces a fairly broad range of reactions, around the fundamental granulomatous process. Similarly, Jones and Campbell, observing only a few cases of *avium*-Battey lymphadenitis in children, found no distinguishing histological feature.[179]

Lesions observed in disseminated mycobacteriosis Group III have rarely resembled the typical lesions of miliary tuberculosis. Since a high proportion of the cases reported have occurred in young children, the possibility of some kind of coexistent immunological incompetency may account for the uncharacteristic lesions.

Pathogenicity for mammals and birds varies widely within the *avium*-Battey complex. Of 10 of 17 strains Marks and Birn had isolated from human tissues and identified as "avian," all were lethal for birds and 6 strains were lethal also in rabbits.[241] The remaining 7 strains, also from human tissue, produced only trivial lesions in fowls. Organisms that Kubin and associates isolated from human tissue in Czechoslovakia were universally lethal for birds and rabbits.[209] Tsukamura *et al.*,[399] using as a measure the number of mycobacterial viable units three weeks after injection into mice, found virulence progressed in the following fashion: avian > human avian > Battey types > Group III isolates from soil. Spontaneous pathogenicity for lower animals has already received notice in Chapter 3.

III. EPIDEMIOLOGY

In the discussion that follows, two or three points deserve emphasis:
(1) Identification of organisms by serotyping is relatively recent, and some
of the most extensive epidemiological investigation antedates this technique. (2) The subject of interest is in fact a ''complex'' of organisms, very
closely related and in many cases indistinguishable by any other method
than serotyping. (3) Even with serotyping, antigens are so similar that only
tests after apparent full absorption serve to separate some varieties.

A. Isolations from the Environment and from Food

As far back as 1935, Stafseth *et al.*[349] demonstrated that eggs derived
from hens infected with *M. avium* contained the organism and thus established one potential pathway by which humans might become infected.
Spontaneous infection of birds, of course, was well known, and it had long
been accepted that various food products for humans might be contaminated with mycobacteria. A chain of infection extending from the barnyard
to poultry to farm animals and, either directly or indirectly, through milk
and eggs to humans was clearly implied. When infection with Battey
organisms assumed so important a place in pulmonary disease in Georgia,
the more recent study of Kubica and his colleagues[206] unmistakably demonstrated a potential source in soil and water.

Three years before, in Michigan, the Mallmans and their associates,[236,237] concerned with the problem of misleading tuberculin tests in
cattle, had similarly demonstrated the presence of avian or closely similar
organisms both in soil and in feed for domestic animals. That similar or
identical organisms produced a scrofulous disease in swine was well established. Obviously, humans who occupied the same contaminated farm
environment underwent some degree of risk. In view of the early studies
reported in Chapter 1, milk seemed to be a vehicle through which atypical
mycobacteria might reach humans.

In 1965, it was reported that 33.9% of samples of unpasteurized milk
taken from refrigerated tankers produced colonies of mycobacteria.[51] The
frequency of positive cultures by season, moreover, corresponded with

Wolinsky's isolations from sputum[431] and with the seasonal distribution of mycobacteria that Atwell and Pratt had observed in gastric washings of both tuberculous and healthy people.[9] Pigmented organisms from raw milk were more numerous with respect to all isolated organisms during the winter months, while nonpigmented ones appeared in samples taken during the summer, an observation supported by cultures of milk sediment from commercial centrifuges.[368,369]

If organisms survived pasteurization, milk as processed might constitute a source of ingested atypical mycobacteria. As early as 1937, Humphriss and his colleagues[170] had demonstrated that methods of pasteurization in use in England at that time allowed viable mycobacteria to pass through to the consumer, and in 1963, Scammon and associates[322] and our laboratory, in a simulation of the slow method of pasteurization, found that atypical mycobacteria survived. Subsequently, Harrington and Karlson[160] simulated both slow and rapid methods in their laboratory with similar results. In all cases, it appeared that the best survivors were pigmented types, but in the experiment of Harrington and Karlson, 12% of nonpigmented strains remained viable. It remained only to show that the standard commercial pasteurization allowed viable mycobacteria to appear in milk. In 1968, it was reported that of 458 samples of packaged milk taken from the shelf, 2.8% contained mycobacteria. Of the 13 strains isolated, 9 proved to be members of Group III.[57]

Throughout these various reports, identification did not go beyond assignment to the *avium*-Battey complex. Serotyping permits a far more accurate and precise mode of identification. Kazda's investigation of "*M. brunense*,"[187] as an example, demonstrated that that organism maintained viability after four hours at 60°. It could be isolated from birds and from water, and when it was injected into chickens, it produced nonspecific tuberculin sensitivity. This organism, subsequently more fully identified not as a species but as serotype "Davis," had produced infection in swine and cattle in the United States and had been isolated from human material in Czechoslovakia[211] and in other parts of Europe.[113,187]

In more specifically human environments, Japanese investigators[393] have recently compared the mycobacterial population of dusts in patients' rooms with the organisms excreted in sputum. *Mycobacterium intracellulare* appeared in 69.6% of Group III isolations from sputum, while it accounted for only 0.5% isolations from dust. Conversely, an organism they called *Mycobacterium nonchromogenicum* furnished 23.5% isolations from dust against only 3% from sputum.

Other sources of infection or colonization to which humans may be exposed have included drinking water[186,211] and several kinds of edible meats.[378] A fascinating recent contribution by Gruft *et al.*[149] has demonstrated the presence of *M. intracellulare* in ocean waters and its aerogenous dispersal by rupture of bubbles of foam. Of much greater significance as a potential source of human infection is ordinary potable water. Goslee and Wolinsky[142] have very recently reported the recovery of 80 strains of *M. gordonae* as well as 47% organisms of the *avium–intracellulare–scrofulaceum* complex. Not only are organisms present, but they appear in numbers, an average of 3.5 strains per sample.

B. Isolations from Animals

Many isolations of Group III organisms have been made from the tissues of both birds and animals. The relationship of such isolates to infection in humans has been demonstrated only in the past six years. Yoder and Schaefer, for example, serotyped 188 strains from birds, cattle, swine and other animals.[444] Of these strains, 31 proved to be Avian I and 127 were Avian II, while 30 were *M. intracellulare* of 8 different serotypes. Of the *intracellulare* strains, only a third were pathogenic for chickens as opposed to 99% for Avian II. Of 128 strains only from cattle, 106 were avian, 16 were *M. intracellulare*, and 6 were uncertain. In England and Wales, infections of birds are very widespread and severe, and all of these infections can be ascribed to Avian I or Avian II, which also accounted for 16 of 17 infections in cattle (retropharyngeal lymph nodes) and 22 of 25 in swine (submandibular nodes).[326] Elsewhere, Schaefer reported that Avian I and Avian II accounted for organisms from all birds and for about half the infections among pigs and cows.[325] At that time, only 20% of strains isolated from humans corresponded to the avian serotypes. Kazda's investigation also establishes Avian II as the principal infectious agent for birds, but he found organisms of this serotype also in samples of water.[187]

Avian tuberculosis may become hematogenous in both sheep and swine.[81] Ordinarily, the infection is less severe and is confined to nodes. One study in the United States in 1938 revealed avian bacilli in tissues of 16 of 32 hogs, but in several instances, organisms have been recovered from nodes in which there were no visible abnormalities.[348] Isolations of avian organisms from pigs were also frequent in France.[367] However, in Australia, when an outbreak of lymphatic disease developed in 50 of 77 pigs, the organism was identified as serotype VI. The same serotype was also found in their feed, water, and litter.[373]

Careful studies of organisms isolated at Lansing, Michigan, demonstrated that avian or avianlike organisms occurred with considerable frequency in the nodes of swine and also in nodes and cutaneous lesions of cattle. Not all strains were pathogenic for chickens, but their injection resulted in hypersensitivity to both avian and mammalian tuberculins. More importantly, it was observed that inoculation into young pigs might or might not result in lesions but that inoculated swine developed reactions to both avian and mammalian tuberculin, and that tissues frequently contained organisms in the absence of detectable lesions.[236,237]

The use of avian and mammalian tuberculin may be undertaken in studies of animal populations, but the results may not necessarily be pertinent. In the case of avian tuberculosis of a young child, Feldman *et al.*[122] found half of the chickens, 30% of the cattle, and two of six swine on the family farm to react to avian antigen. In England, reactions of normal animals to avian tuberculin are common,[283] and unreported studies of a herd in southeast Texas revealed very extensive reaction to avian tuberculin, though none of the reactors subsequently slaughtered exhibited gross lesions.

Variable hypersensitivity, pathological findings, and presence of organisms in pathological or normal tissue have also been reported from Scandinavia,[112] Ireland,[270] and Japan.[395] Horses, as well, have produced positive reactions to avian tuberculin.[200]

C. Human Isolations and Hypersensitivity

Isolations from so many environmental and other sources suggest that humans should be subject to considerable exposure to organisms of the *avium–intracellulare* complex. Furthermore, experience with skin tests in animals suggests that humans may be sensitized even though they present no evidence of disease. Three kinds of information are available to indicate the extent or frequency of exposure to members of this mycobacterial complex: skin tests; isolations from humans who are free of disease; and the appearance of clinical disease in human populations.

1. Skin Tests

The problems of interpretation of the significance of skin tests have received notice in Chapter 3. It is sufficient to summarize that the agent most frequently and extensively employed in the United States has been PPD-B, that it has revealed a much higher prevalence of reactivity in the southeastern part of the country, and that its specificity has been seriously overestimated by some reports. The statement in 1974 of Wijsmuller and Erickson[428] that "the vast majority of reactors did not acquire their sensitivity to PPD-Battey through infections with intracellulare (sic)" appears to be a fair appraisal. However, one should reiterate the difference from sensitivity acquired through the invasion of tissue.

In Britain, the usual antigen employed for nontuberculous sensitization has been avian tuberculin. Reactions are numerous among schoolchildren, but there is evidence, discussed in the general consideration of epidemiology, that these reactions are transitory and variable.

2. Cultures from Healthy People

In Georgia, Edwards and Palmer[107] cultured sputums and saliva from 122 persons over 14 years of age. All had normal roentgenograms of the chest. These cultures produced four strains of Group II organisms, 8 of Group III, and five of Group IV. On two farms, 40% of the adults were found to excrete material containing mycobacteria. In tropical Australia, Kiewiet and Thompson[193] cultured secretions from 290 males whose roentgenograms of the chest were normal. Bronchial secretions produced 22 strains of mycobacteria, of which 20 were organisms belonging to either Group II or Group III. Also in Australia, Singer obtained positive cultures from 30 of 441 pairs of removed tonsils.[337] Of these, 17 strains were identified as Group II and 9 as Group III organisms. In East Anglia, Stewart and associates also studied resected tonsils as well as throat swabbings. In this instance, cultures of tonsils were positive for *avium*-like organisms.[355] The oropharynx, however, is not the only source of mycobacteria among healthy people, for Carruthers and Edwards[45] reported 11 isolations from specimens of urine from people without evidence of disease.

3. Epidemiology of Disease

Since skin tests provide less than specific information and since isolations from healthy people undoubtedly are very frequent without much respect to geography, established cases with evident disease finally provide the most reliable information with respect to epidemiology. Until serotyping becomes a regular part of the identification, even unequivocal disease produces information that is only broadly applicable.

a. Geography. From Table 10-1, it is obvious that infection with *avium*-Battey strains is widespread. Lack of reports from other areas, however, does not signify absence of disease but may indicate a lack of facilities, failure to collect a large series of properly verified cases, or different modes of reporting. Moreover, the distribution of serotypes is somewhat selective geographically. Schaefer's report[325] states that Avian I and Avian II were much more common among isolates from Wales, Denmark, and Czechoslovakia than among isolates of American origin. In Japan, this country,[318] and Australia,[308] other than avian serotypes account for most of the human infections.

b. Age. The study of Ahn *et al.*[3] (though not reflecting distribution of serotypes) provides an excellent comparison of age between patients with infections due to *M. kansasii* and those with infections due to *M. intracellulare*. Since the only restriction with respect to selection was that of political boundaries, the two sets of patients appear to be comparable. Texas patients with *M. intracellulare* infection averaged about 10 years older (mean 58 years) than the group with mycobacteriosis kansasii. These figures agree well with a mean of 56 years for cases in Georgia[74] and of 54 years for cases reported from Wisconsin.[311]

c. Sex. In reports from Japan (see Table 10-1), the male:female ratio is 2:1, while in larger series from America, the proportion is 7:3 and 4:1. In Australian series, the proportion of males is even greater.

d. Race. In those studies in which there appears to be little selection

TABLE 10-1
Features of Pulmonary Mycobacteriosis Caused by Group III Organisms

Report	Source	% Male	Age	% of all atypical	Remarks
74	Georgia	71	56 mean	100	1.5% admis.
224	Florida	chiefly	40–60	100	2% admis.
295	Missouri	75	50%>54	75	
287	U.S. South (VA)	100	75%>50	?	
443	Houston (VA)	100	49%>50	?	
189	Utah (VA)	100	84%>50	75	
123	Denver	76	52 mean	40	4.2% admis.
3	Texas	72	58 mean	32	
61	Dallas	80	"Middle-aged"	21.7	
311	Milwaukee	78	54 mean	90	
356	Boston		53	83	
414	Connecticut	93	"Older"	73	0.9% admis.
139	London	80		27	1.3% admis.
134	France			44	0.9% cultures
	England–Wales	chiefly			1.5% admis.
310	British Columbia		"Older"	74	
45	Western Australia	80	"Older"	98	5% admis.
124	New South Wales			62	
397	Japan			98	2.6% admis.
441	Japan	67			

from an ethnically diverse population, incidence by race appears to be about proportional to ethnic distribution.

   e. Occupational and Social Factors. Infections with serotypes Avian I and II appear to be particularly associated with rural life and with mining, according to studies in Wales.[326] In other areas, without regard to serotype, various strains of *M. intracellulare* appear in disease of people with rural residence (see Table 10-1).

   f. Associated Disease. Infection with varieties of the *avium*-Battey complex seems to be closely associated with silicosis or anthracosis.[133,183,326,414] Other chronic pulmonary disease has been recognized as a factor in non-miners.[182,240,310] The analysis of Ahn and coauthors[3] indicates that infection with Group III pathogens occurs in individuals who exhibit restrictive defects (there is only an impression, without assurance, that fibrosis preceded the infection). In the cases Yeager and Raleigh studied,[443] however, obstructive disease was present in 56%.

    g. Familial Occurrence. With very extensive experience of the disease among patients in Georgia, Corpe asserted that he had never encountered disease in two members of the same family.[74] Most reports have agreed with this statement.[221] Engbaek, however, encountered three cases of fatal disseminated avian infection in a mother and her two daughters,[110] while Van Zeben encountered two cases of cervical adenitis in siblings.[406] In a study of familial contacts of a patient with severe avian infection, Crompton *et al.*[82] found 66.6% of the contacts reactive to an avian sensitin, with a comparative rate of 37.5% for control families. Prather *et al.*[295] also found a clustering of sensitivity and cultures in families of probands, the children with an increased rate of reaction to PPD-B and a few adults without disease but with secretions containing organisms. It should be pointed out with respect to studies of families, however, that clusters of sensitivity or of positive cultures may signify as much a common environment as the possibility of person-to-person transmission.

    h. Other Factors. In the study of Prather *et al.,* there was clearly a peak of incidence during the winter months, an observation of some interest in connection with other observations of seasonal effects on isolations of mycobacteria. Other factors may be involved, but the unavailability of serotyping in so many reports prevents any precise delineation of them.

IV. CLINICAL FEATURES

A. "Primary" Infection

    In the series studied by Prather *et al.,*[295] one child exhibited a pulmonary lesion that might be interpreted as primary pulmonary mycobacteriosis. In a single instance, Singer encountered an *avium*-Battey organism among cultures of mediastinal nodes of patients who met with sudden death. In 48 autopsies of patients who died after treatment in hospital, no mediastinal nodes were found to contain organisms.[337] Aside from these two instances, there is no evidence to suggest a primary pulmonary infection resembling that of *M. tuberculosis*. Evidence that "primary" infection occurs in the oropharyx appears in the discussion of cervical lymphadenitis in Section IV.A. in Chapter 8.

B. Pulmonary Disease in Adults

1. Symptoms

None of Corpe's patients had temperatures higher than 100°.[74] In the series of Kamat *et al.*,[183] 75% were symptomatic, but the symptoms for the most part were even milder than those produced by *M. kansasii*. These authors pointed out, however, that hemoptysis is more common than in patients with tuberculosis. Most writers agree that infection with strains of the *avium*-Battey complex produces relatively little change in health, particularly in that many patients have preexisting pulmonary disease.

2. Physical Findings

Findings upon physical examination are few, as in other pulmonary mycobacterioses, and their interpretation is frequently clouded by the presence of other disease of the lung.

3. Laboratory Findings

The usual procedures furnish little other than negative information, with the exception of acid-fast stains of the sputum. Organisms usually appear to be somewhat shorter than *M. tuberculosis,* and bipolar distribution of dye may be observed. (It should be remembered that antimicrobial therapy affects the appearance of the tubercle bacillus and that variability of morphology of mycobacteria is to be expected: at most, microscopic examination can produce only presumptive information.) The diagnosis depends entirely upon cultures and bacteriological identification, with serotyping greatly to be desired.

4. Roentgenographic Examination

In a study of patients in a Veterans Administration hospital, Yeager and Raleigh[443] found that 50% had multiple cavities, although theses were unilateral in about half. In the series of Lewis *et al.*,[224] cavities were observed in 78% of all cases; in Corpe's series,[74] 50% were classified as "far advanced," a designation formerly used to signify a single cavity greater than 4 cm in diameter, or a number of small cavities, without respect to distribution. Pleural effusions were observed in approximately 2–3% of roentgenograms, though the presence of fluid does not necessarily indicate that it resulted from mycobacterial infection.

One Japanese group[398] and a report from Western Australia maintained that there were no distinguishing features in the roentgenograms of the chest. However, Tsukamura[391] noted absence of pericavitary infiltration as a striking feature of *avium*-Battey disease, while to Tsai *et al.*[383] small nodulations, as opposed to soft, fluffy infiltrations, appeared to be significant of infection by mycobacteria other than *M. tuberculosis*. At best, differences can be only suggestive.

5. Differential Diagnosis

Pulmonary disease caused by strains of this complex require differentiation from tuberculosis and from pulmonary histoplasmosis. Repeated sputum cultures, preferably at least three with growth greater than 100 colonies in each, provide the only reliable differentiation from tuberculosis and other mycobacteriosis of the lung.

Many epidemiological and clinical features are common to histoplasmosis and *avium*-Battey mycobacteriosis. The clinical course and the roentgenograms may also be very similar. Cultures of sputum supported by serological tests for histoplasmosis are essential.

C. Disease of Lymph Nodes

The description of lymphadenitis in Chapter 8 applies equally to lymphadenitis caused by strains of the *avium*-Battey complex. Although organisms of this complex produce disease of lymph nodes less frequently than does *M. scrofulaceum,* in some areas the infection is by no means rare. In Western Australia, 9 of 12 infections of cervical lymph nodes resulted from organisms of Group III.[45] In the study of Schaefer *et al.,*[326] 4 cases of pediatric lymphadenitis resulted from infection with *M. avium,* while 12 were caused by members of the Battey group (serotypes Davis, Yandle, and VI). In New South Wales, 3 of 4 cases of cervical lymphadenitis were caused by nonchromogenic organisms, as were 2 of 6 cases in the Netherlands.[406] In England, only one of 15 cultures isolated from lymph nodes of children proved to be a Battey-type organism. In one study in Texas, two nonchromogenic organisms were isolated among 13 other atypical mycobacteria that had produced pediatric lymphadenitis.[30]

According to a review by Kubin *et al.,*[210] all cases of cervical lymphadenopathy attributed to genuine avian types have appeared in Europe, and particularly in Germany. In these patients, the narrowly restricted range of age (about one to five years) observed in the United States and Canada does not hold, since the disease has frequently appeared in older children and even in adults.

The range of clinical and pathological findings resembles those of *M. scrofulaceum.* The treatment consists of excision of nodes and of sinus tracts, if any have formed.

D. Cutaneous Disease

Organisms of the *avium*-Battey complex rarely give rise to lesions of the skin. In widely disseminated, hematogenous disease, Koenig *et al.*[198] observed a serpiginous, plaquelike infiltration of the skin, and in a 27-month-old child, Volini and associates[411] found a widespread macular rash. Yakovac *et al.*[440] also observed nodular lesions of the scalp in a young child with disseminated disease. In an older patient, also with extensive dissemination, Schachter[323] observed a deep ulcer of the leg, which upon biopsy revealed granulomatous infiltrations and acid-fast bacilli.

More typically, antigen antibody reaction occurred in one of Engbaek's cases.[110] The disease in this instance was limited to a single lobe of the lungs, but erythema nodosum appeared soon after the onset of the infection.

The case reported by Schmidt *et al.*[329] seems to be the only instance of primary infection of the skin. Some two weeks after injury, nodular swelling took place in an area of minor abrasion. After a second elapse of two weeks, the nodulation underwent necrosis and resulted in an ulcer about 2 cm in diameter.

E. Bones and Soft Tissues

Except in disseminated disease with widespread osteomyelitis (see Table 10-2), isolated involvement of bones and soft tissues is relatively unusual. In the review by Schaefer and others,[326] there was a single instance of "ganglion" affecting the tendon sheath at the wrist. The experience of Kelly and associates[190] included six instances of isolated infections of tendon sheaths, three patients with infections of the knee joint, and two patients with infection of bursae. Since two-thirds of the strains isolated were nonchromogenic, some of these lesions unquestionably resulted from infections by members of the *avium*-Battey complex. The child reported by Levine[223] had bilateral cellulitis involving the orbits of the eyes.

Dechairo *et al.*[92] described infection of the hip joint, by *M. triviale*, ordinarily considered a nonpathogen, but evidence for osseous disease was lacking. A boy of five years was seen in Dallas when he presented with a large cystlike lesion in the lower end of the femur. During three months, the area of rarefaction enlarged greatly and perforated into the knee joint. The synovium contained a granulomatous and purulent process, and the joint was filled with purulent fluid. Cultures of synovium and fluid each produced a nonchromogenic mycobacterium.[47]

Other cases of osteomyelitis caused by strains of Battey organisms have been aspects of disseminated disease. These have somewhat resembled staphylococcal osteomyelitis, though the evolution is slower. The periosteum is elevated, and pus frequently dissects its way to the surface and produces multiple draining sinuses. About half of the organisms involved have been clearly identified as avian types,[91,110,240] while others have been various serotypes of the *avium*-Battey complex or have not been typed.[404,411,440]

Surgical treatment in the cases reported by Kelly *et al.* consisted of removal of synovial membranes, tendon sheaths, or bursae.[190] When pus is accessible, it should be drained, regardless of the fact that persistent

TABLE 10-2
Disseminated *Avium*-Battery Mycobacteriosis[a]

Report	Age	Organism[b]	Bone	Other lesions	Remarks
101	5 yrs.	III	0	Meningitis; lymph nodes	
84	34 mos.	I.C.	0	Specific colitis	Polyserositis; Gaucher's disease
404	2 yrs.	III	Multiple	Liver, lungs, spleen, nodes	Cortisone treatment
440	19 mos.	III	Multiple	Nodes	
247	71 yrs.	III	0	Liver, spleen, bone marrow	Leukopenia, purpura
110	Adult	Av.	Multiple	0	
411	27 mos.	III	Multiple	Liver, spleen	43,000 WBC; 11% eos.; Letterer–Siwe pattern
91	19 yrs.	Av. I	Multiple	0	7% eos.
210-I	25 yrs.	Av.	0	Nodes, meninges	Sarcoidosis pattern, leukopenia
198	62 yrs.	III	0	Liver, spleen, nodes, marrow	36,000 WBC
60	5½ yrs.	III	Multiple	0	
330	12 yrs.	Av.	Multiple	Spleen, liver, serous cavities	
326	—	I.C.	0	Miliary	
323 3 cases	Adults	III	0	Diffuse lymphatic disease	
415	63 yrs.	Av. I	0	Liver, spleen, nodes, lungs	Leukemia? Reticulum-cell sarcoma
214	—	Av. I	0	Liver, bone marrow	Leukopenia
117	63 yrs.	III	0	Lungs, bone marrow; kidney?	
320	Adult	I.C.	0	Prostate, meninges, retroperitoneal nodes	

[a] In chronological order of report.
[b] Serotype indicated by Av. I or I.C.

sinuses may remain. Extensive removal of necrotic bone is impossible in disseminated disease with many sites of osteomyelitis. In the management of these problems, effective antimicrobial therapy represents the most suitable treatment.

Diagnosis of infection with these organisms depends rather on culture than on histological study of tissue. Quite a number of reported instances of disseminated osteomyelitis have revealed histological changes that did not strongly suggest a mycobacterial etiology.[84,223,411] This departure from the expected reaction is particularly common among young children (see Table 10-2).

F. Genitourinary Tract

It is important to note that isolations of nonchromogenic mycobacteria from urine have occurred in the absence of any demonstrable disease or symptoms. Carruthers and Edwards,[45] for example, obtained 11 positive cultures of routine specimens of urine. On the other hand, in widely disseminated disease, the examination postmortem has often revealed either no disease or only minor lesions.

Isolated disease, apparently restricted to the genitourinary tract, has occurred. The patient of Faber *et al.*[116] offered as a primary complaint hematuria. Retrograde pyelography demonstrated only slight irregularity in the left superior calyx. After a partial nephrectomy, tissue revealed zones of epithelioid cells. Organisms were cultured from the resected tissue.

Tsai *et al.*[383] encountered a problem of pyuria in a patient with pulmonary disease as well. Both urine and sputum produced mycobacteria of Group III. Retrograde pyelography demonstrated an abscess connecting with the upper pole of one renal pelvis.

Newman's patient[265] complained of dysuria and the urine contained pus. Cystoscopy and intravenous pyelography failed to reveal abnormality, but retrograde pyelography demonstrated blunting of the calyces and a hydroureter on the left side. Ureteral catheterization produced urine containing very many acid-fast bacilli. In the course of three months, the disease progressed rapidly and the function of the left kidney ceased. After nephrectomy, histological examination revealed dilatation, hydronephrosis, and whorled fibrous tissue that replaced the renal cortex. Here and there were areas of Langhans giant cells, with patchy central necrosis.

The patient of Pergament *et al.*[284] had end-stage disease at the time of consultation. At the lower pole of the left kidney, it was possible to demonstrate an abscess, with evidence of calcification in the wall. Drainage of the abscess resulted in identification of Group III organisms, and further urological examination disclosed a small, contracted bladder and a nonfunctioning left kidney. At nephrectomy, the left kidney was found to be entirely destroyed and its structure replaced by dense fibrous tissue.

It is evident that while the discovery of Group III mycobacteria in the urine may not be associated with any disease, it is essential to carry out complete examination. The cases cited represent progression from the earliest detectable abnormality to total destruction, and at least one of them confirms that progression may take place fairly rapidly.

Treatment has consisted of standard urological procedures such as were applied to renal lesions caused by *M. tuberculosis*. Infections of the kidney caused by Group III organisms apparently have not often been managed by antimicrobial therapy. It might be anticipated that some success might result from a regimen carefully designed for the susceptibility of the particular strain, but only if the lesion is a relatively limited one.

G. Disseminated Disease

Reference to Table 10-2 demonstrates that dissemination of organisms of the *avium*-Battey group presents some features different from those of other disseminated atypical mycobacterioses. Bone appears to be much more often involved, but it is well worth noting that while every serotyped instance of osseous disease revealed a strain of avian organisms, not one has been serotyped as a member of the Battey group. Dissemination in spleen, liver, lungs, and lymph nodes occurs as might be expected of any mycobacterium. Close reading of the report, however, makes it seem very probable that five cases appear to have originated in the abdomen, with massive disease in mesenteric and retroperitoneal lymph nodes.[84,210,320,330,411] The first manifestation of one of these was a mass about the head of the pancreas. Another striking feature is that these infections are much more frequent in childhood than are other disseminated mycobacterioses.[320] Peripheral leukocyte counts are frequently quite elevated (25,000–45,000), and eosinophiles appear in high percentage (5–10%) for such a degree of leukocytosis. The striking difference in age may account for the differences observed, since *M. kansasii* most often has disseminated in patients with pancytopenia or leukopenia who fall into an older range of age.

V. SUSCEPTIBILITY AND TREATMENT

A. Tests *in Vitro*

One of the features that first called renewed attention to atypical mycobacteria was their relative resistance to concentrations of isoniazid that would inhibit most strains of *M. tuberculosis*. There was also resistance to PAS. To streptomycin, however, the resistance was usually less striking, and a good many strains were susceptible to 3.6 μg/ml. However, it became apparent that strains rapidly acquire almost total resistance to this substance. Strains have varied in susceptibility,[168,332] as might be anticipated from the numerous serotypes included within the group.

Resistance to these primary antituberculosis drugs led to exploration of susceptibility to other antimicrobials. Birn *et al.*[27] found nearly all their avian strains to be sensitive to cycloserine but resistant to ethionamide, even at concentrations of 40 μg/ml. Hawkins and McClean,[163] without reference to serotypes, found most strains of Group III susceptible to cycloserine at concentrations of between 1.0 and 50 μg/ml. Engbaek *et al.*, also working with several varieties, over three-fourths of which were serotype Avian II, reported almost all strains susceptible to cycloserine.[113]

Availability of rifampin has somewhat improved the possibility of satisfactory treatment. Tsukamura[390] discovered that most American strains of *M. intracellulare* were susceptible, while Japanese and Rhodesian varieties were not. Resistance of a strain to this drug seemed to correlate with its ability to use butanol as a sole source of carbon and to grow at 45°. The studies of Rynearson *et al.*[316] apparently demonstrated that opaque colonies of Group III organisms were more susceptible to rifampin than translucent ones.

Other possibly effective antimicrobials have also received attention. In 1961, Virtanen found that a majority of atypical mycobacteria were susceptible to kanamycin and to sulfadiazine.[409] Of 41 Group III strains, 17 were also susceptible to erythromycin, as also reported in the same year by Guy and Chapman,[157] who found most of their strains, derived from Runyon's Battey pack, to be susceptible at 5 μg/ml, while a few were inhibited by 1.0 μg/ml. Other support for the use of sulfonamides has come from the work of Lewis *et al.*[224] (sulfasoxazole) and Birn and associates,[27] with particular respect to *M. avium,* provisional species I.

A current, very interesting report found that benzyl penicillin inhibited 42 of 43 strains of *M. intracellulare* at 10 μg/ml. However, though the tests were definite *in vitro*, the usefulness of this substance could not be confirmed when it was applied to the control of disease in animals. Another drug that has elicited some recent interest is B-663, now available in Europe as lamprene.[268] It is effective *in vitro* at approximately the same concentration as isoniazid. Capreomycin has been used as an injectable when organisms are resistant to attainable concentrations of streptomycin.

B. Trials *in Vivo*

On account of the great variety of organisms included in this complex, as well as the difficulty in producing a satisfactory model of disease in animals, there have been relatively few studies. The recent report of Rynearson *et al.* on the treatment of infection in animals with *M. intracellulare* makes it appear that a combination of streptomycin and rifampin should be the most effective combination available.[316]

C. Experience in Human Disease

Reports of the treatment of large series have almost uniformly presented rather dismal results (see Table 10-3). All of these reports antedate treatment with rifampin, and the basis of most regimens has been INH–PAS–SM, with some substitutions. With antimycobacterial drugs alone, the conversion rate seems to range around 40–50%, unless surgery is employed. When surgery is available to the patient, sputum conversion may reach as high as 60–75%. Even in the face of negative sputum, however, a relapse of about 20% can be anticipated in the following five

TABLE 10-3
Results of Treatment, *Avium*-Battey Infection

Report	No.	Sputum neg.	Surg.	Results
224	68	43	38	17 d., 11 of disease
311	82	34	18	6 relapses
443	45	50%	42%	20% progressed
				19.6% relapsed
74	NS	75% c surg.	NS	NS
182	63	30/52	NS	31 no change or
				worse (X ray)
398	64	31% c surg.	8	NS

years. All cited sources agree that if the distribution of disease and pulmonary function permit, resection constitutes the best assurance of cure.

(Surgery, however, presents its own problems. Law,[218] reviewing the experience of VA hospitals in resection for atypical mycobacterial disease, found 26 surgical complications in 91 resections of varying extent. However, only 8 of these might be considered important: they considered of 5 bronchopleural fistulas, one empyema [nonmycobacterial], and 2 postoperative spreads of disease.)

Disseminated disease in humans may be considered a better model against which to test the efficacy of a therapeutic combination than any model that can be contrived in small animals. Table 10-4 presents available information—fortunately rather more complete than can be obtained from larger series—in these special and very threatening conditions. Since many patients with disseminated infection failed to survive, it is evident that some factor or combination of factors was beneficial in the cases in Table 10-4. The numbers of both types are too few for the matching of cases, and observations at this time are highly tentative. Two of these survivors received rifampin, and one of these, though the youngest, was apparently infected by the least virulent organism. Three patients, all severely ill, received erythromycin. Without undue inference, it appears that severely ill patients might well be treated with both these agents.

On the basis of all the evidence available at this time, the best combination for routine treatment of pulmonary and most other nonthreatening mycobacteriosis caused by Group III organisms seems to be rifampin, streptomycin, and cycloserine. Ethionamide is probably of little value,

TABLE 10-4
Antimicrobials Employed in Successful Treatment of
Disseminated Group III Disease

Report	Organism	Sites	Drugs	Results
214[a]	Avian I	Marrow, liver	INH–RMP	Recovered
92	*M. triviale*	Hip joint	INH–RMP Erythromycin	Recovered
91	Avian I	Mult. bones.	SM–INH Erythromycin	Recovered[b]
60	"Battey"	Mult. bones.	SM–ETH Lincomycin	Recovered[c]
67	Avian II	Gen. visceral	EMB, gentamycin; erythromycin; pentamidine	Died[d]

[a]This patient originally suffered some process marked by severe depression of the bone marrow and leukopenia.
[b]After first treatment, this patient remained well for three years and then suffered relapse. He improved upon retreatment but after six months suffered a second relapse.
[c]Treatment at first was entirely successful, but after a year, disease recurred. Retreatment was successful.
[d]The course was one of improvement for a few months and then worsening. This continued for many months.

though ethambutol may be effective against some strains. Because many Group III organisms possess an amidase for pyrazinamide,[33] that drug would probably have no place. Erythromycin 2 g daily might be required as a result of toxicity or other difficulty. Since sulfonamides are usually well tolerated, it is worthwhile to obtain susceptibility of the individual strain to these substances, while the observation of an effect of benzyl penicillin *in vitro* would justify its trial along with some of the more common antimycobacterial agents in problems of life-threatening disease.

VI. OTHER GROUP III INFECTIONS

In Table 10-4 appear the basic facts in regard to a young child who developed septic arthritis of the hip, with *M. triviale* as the apparent agent. Cianciulli[63] has reported the case of a 21-year-old white female, apparently previously quite healthy, who developed miliary tuberculosis, confirmed by culture of the organism from a hepatic biopsy. Hardly had she recovered from this infection, when she developed equally widespread disseminated disease caused by *M. terrae,* which was cultured from the liver, the bone marrow, and the urine. Recovery occurred spontaneously.

There is little doubt that in the course of time, other infections caused by these "nonpathogenic" members of Group III may occur. However, it is very unlikely that they will play other than an opportunistic and occasional role, and the occurrence of such infections does not refute the basic opinion that they are rarely agents of disease.

It is obvious, in view of the unpredictable susceptibilities of such organisms, that each isolate may call for a different combination of drugs and that in many cases recovery may occur if the patient has no permanent impairment of his immunological system.

11

Mycobacterium xenopi

Mycobacterium xenopi was first isolated by Schwabacher from a nodular lesion on the back of a frog (*Xenopus laevis,* the South African clawed toad). After isolating the organism, he was able to reintroduce it into a similar animal and reproduce the lesion.[332] (Many references use the term *xenopei,* the form Schwabacher originally chose.)

I. BACTERIOLOGY

Contrary to Schwabacher's supposition, *M. xenopi* does not grow well at 24° but for best growth requires 43–45°.[100,108,147,155] On cornmeal agar, colonies exhibit branching filaments, but on Loewenstein–Jensen, the colonies are butyrous, originally buff but gradually manifesting pigmentation from lemon-yellow to orange-yellow.[100,108] The three-day or four-day aryl-sulfatase test is positive, as are the urease and catalase tests. The organism reduces nitrate to nitrite.[332]

In spite of its pigmentation, *M. xenopi* is regarded as a member of Runyon's Group III. It is virulent for birds, and serotyping places it very near Schaefer's Avian I,[172] but it cross-reacts also with antibodies against *M. intracellulare.*

II. PATHOLOGY AND PATHOGENESIS

Since identification of the organism has been rather inconsistent, descriptions of the pathological processes resulting from infection with *M. xenopi* are very limited. Engbaek *et al.*[114] stated only that the changes they found were consistent with tuberculosis. In the mesenteric nodes of swine, Jarnagin and associates[172] found "multiple coalescing granulomas with necrotic centers, surrounded by granulation tissue composed mostly of epithelioid cells." Mycobacteria in the center of granulomas appear in spleens and livers of chickens 60 days after inoculation.

III. EPIDEMIOLOGY

A. Lower Animals

Except for Schwabacher's isolation, the organism is not known to affect cold-blooded animals. Isolation from the lymph nodes of swine has been mentioned.

B. Environment

Mycobacterium xenopi has been found in water from both hot and cold taps[40] and from two hot water generators set at 42°, the optimum temperature for growth.[147] Search of other environmental sources, including pigeon droppings, razor scrapings, tooth brushes, and tooth powder, failed to result in isolations of this organism.[40]

C. Geography

Isolations and identifications of *M. xenopi* have been much more frequent in northwestern Europe than in America.[155] In Denmark, *M. xenopi* accounts for 10% of all atypical mycobacteria,[114] while in the United Kingdom, residents of the south and east coasts of England and

Wales have provided most of the isolates. Stewart *et al.*,[355] working in Norfolk, cultured 6 strains of *M. xenopi* from 789 pairs of removed tonsils, 60% of all strains of atypical mycobacteria isolated from this source.

D. Sex

Among 20 patients in whom *M. xenopi* was judged the etiological agent of disease, Marks and Schwabacher[244] found that 16 were males. No other comparative figures have been found.

IV. CLINICAL FEATURES

The clinical course, so far as it has received attention, has not differed appreciably from that produced by other atypical mycobacteria. It may be of some significance that one of the patients described by Engbaek and associates[114] apparently suffered from a specific epididymitis caused by *M. xenopi*. Further, 5 of 50 isolations from human material were derived from urine,[244] though the authors considered that the organisms had not produced detectable genitourinary disease.

In view of the readiness with which *M. xenopi* may be isolated from tap water, it is obvious that occasional isolations from human material of only a few colonies must be regarded with considerable reservation, since nebulization of organisms into the atmosphere of laboratories might lead to the contamination of media.

V. SUSCEPTIBILITY AND TREATMENT

Schwabacher reported that his original strain was susceptible to INH 1 μg/ml and also to streptomycin and PAS. Subsequent tests of other strains have resulted in variable results. The strains Boisvert[31] examined were mostly susceptible to streptomycin and viomycin but not to ethambutol, pyrazinamide, or PAS. The strains Doyle *et al.*[100] tested were inhibited by INH, by streptomycin, and also by erythromycin 15μg; dimethylchlorotetracycline 5 μg; and penicillin G 10 units. Danish strains have been reported susceptible to viomycin, streptomycin, cycloserine, and ethionamide but resistant to INH and PAS at concentrations achievable in patients.[114]

Clinical observations have been too few to permit sound conclusions as to regimens of choice, and since the infection in humans is characteristically rather benign, one may await the result of the susceptibility tests before commencing therapy.[100,108,244]

PART V

THE RAPIDLY GROWING MYCOBACTERIA

12

Mycobacterium fortuitum (with *M. chelonei, M. borstelense,* and *M. abscessus*)

I. NOMENCLATURE

These several organisms are considered under the same heading both for convenience and as a result of uncertainty. Bacteriologists have not reached complete agreement as to the exact relationship among them. Clinical studies and reports often antedate the separation of *M. abscessus* but present infections that seem clearly to result from the organism now known by that name. *Mycobacterium borstelense* and *M. chelonei* appear as organisms in a number of reports but are thought (see below) to be identical with *M. abscessus.*

II. BACTERIOLOGY

All organisms included in the present discussion produce full growth in four or five days. For other biochemical features, consult Table 2-4.

In Stanford's view, *M. abscessus* differs from *M. fortuitum* in failure to reduce nitrate or acetamide and in inability to utilize lactate.[171] Tsukamura,[389] using a battery of enzymatic and biochemical tests, found that *M. abscessus* resembled *M. fortuitum* in 86% of the characters he studied and resembled *M. borstelense* in 80% of traits. Conversely, *M. borstelense* resembled *M. fortuitum* in only 66% of characters. Marks and Szulga[245] attempted to distinguish "pathogenic" from "nonpathogenic" Group IV strains by thin-layer chromatography of their lipids but were unable to accomplish this undertaking. This technique did succeed in establishing that among the 17 strains they tested, 4 differed widely from the lipid patterns of classical *M. fortuitum*. Inman and associates[171] concluded that their serological methods clearly differentiated *M. abscessus* from *M. fortuitum*.

III. PATHOLOGY

A. The Lungs

The following discussion encounters the same handicap with respect to gross pathology as has already been discussed. Several descriptions are from resected lobes and some of the observations that might have been made at the operating table are therefore unavailable to the pathologist. Extent and character of pleural reaction receives little notice. Lungs have presented variable morphological changes, ranging from consolidation or atelectasis to extensive cavitation and suppuration.

B. Skin and Subcutaneous Tissue

A somewhat painful deep lump occurs at the site of injury or injection. After a time, the lesion may undergo suppuration and eventually form persistent draining sinuses. Other lesions seem gradually to subside without requiring surgical drainage and eventually to produce firm masses of fibrosis in deep subcutaneous or muscular tissue.

C. The Cornea

After an injury to the cornea, the margins of the lesion gradually thicken, the entire cornea becomes injected, and opacities appear, especially centering at the site of entry. In the majority of local cases, a metal fragment has been the provoking foreign body.

D. Other Tissues

Other sites are so rarely involved that descriptions cannot be regarded as helpful or characteristic.

E. Histology

The microscopic appearance of lesions that result from *M. fortuitum* or *M. abscessus* has varied from caseating granuloma rather closely resembling tuberculosis[62] to simple suppuration, necrosis, and nonspecific granulation[159,171] with no evidence of tubercle formation. The general impression from the literature is that more superficial infections, such as those that result from inoculation, are predominantly suppurative, while pulmonary lesions and infections of other deep structures exhibit considerably more tuberculoid structures. In the case of lungs, proximity of the sites of granuloma to lipid has been observed,[13,154] an association that creates some doubt with respect to the relative contribution of the lipid or the organisms to the lesion.

Lesions of the cornea are basically suppurative and are marked by the formation of microabscesses in the strata of the cornea.[448]

Injection of *M. abscessus* into mice produces characteristic lesions, consisting of abscesses of the kidney and miliary abscesses of the brain.[19,171] Before the animals succumb, they rather constantly exhibit "spinning disease," a form of ataxia resulting from a microabscess of the inner ear.

IV. CLINICAL MANIFESTATIONS

A. Superficial Abscesses

A few days after injection of some substance, a tender, warm, and firm mass may be palpated underneath the skin. Subsequently, the process may resolve very slowly or may eventually require incision, after which a persistent sinus forms. Drainage may be intermittent for as long as 18 months or more.[171] The usual locations are over the deltoid muscles, in the buttocks, or in the lateral aspect of the thighs.

The nature of the substance injected seems to be of little moment. Outbreaks of abscesses have occurred after vaccination for influenza,[274] and sporadic cases have appeared after injection of penicillin,[66] insulin, BCG or an iron compound,[19] and histamine.[171] In the very extensive outbreak reported by Owen and associates, a diligent search for the source of infection failed to reveal any break in technique or infection of the injected substance.[174] An iron spike,[131] wounds sustained in battle, thorns, and even surgical wounds[159] have introduced or prepared the way for infection with *M. fortuitum* or *M. abscessus*.

B. Pulmonary Disease

In 1962, Hartwig *et al.*[161] reported isolation of *M. fortuitum* from the sputums of 43 patients. In most instances, only a single specimen produced the organisms, but from 3 patients, cultures resulted in isolations on two or more occasions, and the authors conjectured that in such situations, in the absence of other known pathogenic agents, *M. fortuitum* might have to be considered as the infecting agent. In a similar review of bacteriological isolations in 1973, Awe *et al.*[10] reported isolations of *M. fortuitum* from sputums of 56 patients. In the case of 35 individuals, these findings had occurred as only a few colonies on one or two occasions; in these, the authors felt reasonably certain the organisms played no significant role as an agent of disease. From 21 individuals, however, isolations of the organisms occurred repeatedly and in heavy growth; in this group, the situation was less obvious. One had to consider either a persistent colonization of previously damaged lungs or outright invasion by a supposed "nonpathogenic" organism.

The report of Gacad and Massaro admirably illustrates the difficulties that involve pathogenesis.[129] They isolated *M. fortuitum* repeatedly in two of three patients with ankylosing spondylitis and abnormal pulmonary roentgenograms. In one instance, the organism eventually disappeared from the sputum, but not as a consequence of any treatment. The other patient succumbed, and post mortem examination revealed extensive fibrosis and cavitation, with associated characteristic tuberculoid granulomas. In the judgment of these authors, however, the fibrosis and cavitation for the most part preceded the infection with *M. fortuitum*.

Not only does preexisting disease play some role in infection with *M. fortuitum*, but concomitant injury by other material may permit invasion of an organism that is rarely pathogenic. The patient of Guest *et al.*[154] was found to have aspirated mineral oil, and apparently the mineral oil granulomas existed side by side with cavitation and fibrosis that seemed to result from the acid-fast organism. In the patient reported by Nicholson and Sevier,[266] there was a long history of chronic obstructive pulmonary disease associated with abuse of ethanol. Regurgitation and aspiration seemed to play a possible part in pathogenesis, although when the lower lobe was resected, the primary finding was a 5-cm cavity surrounded by fibrosis and scattered areas of caseating necrosis.

In the report of Bannerjee and associates,[13] there appeared to be interplay among adjuvant material, suppression of immunity, and infection with *M. fortuitum*. The patient was a middle-aged woman with achalasia of the esophagus. In the course of management, she received 40 units of corticotropin twice weekly. Roentenograms revealed gradually progressive fibrosis and consolidation of both lower lobes. After six months, the patient died, and autopsy revealed dense confluent bronchopneumonia with many areas that contained lipids. Acid-fast organisms were present in abundance throughout.

Other impairments of defense mechanisms appear in the cause of Chusid *et al.*[62] Their patient, a young while male, developed pleuritic pain, severe sweats, and a high, spiking fever. Pleural fluid contained *M. fortuitum*, which seemed to have involved the pleura by contiguous spread from a paraspinal abscess and osteomyelitis of a vertebral body. Though no organisms were recovered from the abscess, it was lined by caseating granulomatous tissue.

C. Disseminated Infection

Two patients who had received renal homografts and very intensive immunosuppressive therapy developed widespread infections due to *M. abscessus*. In one patient, the dissemination was manifest as multiple sites of osteomyelitis and numerous subcutaneous abscesses. In the other, infection was limited to numerous subcutaneous abscesses, including one that arose in the mammary gland. It is important to note that the sites were entirely independent of areas in which injections had been given and that the organisms unquestionably were blood-borne.

D. Corneal Infection

For several years, the Department of Ophthalmology at the University of Texas Southwestern Medical School has encountered cases of corneal infection following some type of penetrating injury; most often a fragment of metal from some type of machining process has been involved. In spite of prompt removal of the foreign body, if it is still present, the wound fails to heal, and after a few days purulent drainage begins. The entire cornea becomes injected and opacity develops around the thickened edges of the original site of injury. An organism identified only as *M. fortuitum* has been present in great numbers in the discharge.

A very similar type of corneal inflammation was reported by Wunsch and associates[438] when infection developed in a corneal graft. Zimmerman *et al.*[448] reported two cases of infection after injury. Apparently, infection of the cornea by *M. fortuitum* occurs with appreciable frequency. To the degree that proper repair after injury fails to develop and purulent discharge occurs, smears and cultures for acid-fast bacilli—in addition to the search for more usual organisms—are essential.

V. TREATMENT

A. Subcutaneous Abscesses

The principal treatment has consisted of hot soaks followed by surgical drainage.[43] The rate of healing varies considerably: Clapper[66] observed that following incision, a deep abscess of the buttock continued to drain for as long as two months, and longer periods of infection have occurred, particularly if there happened to be multiple sites.[171] In chronic, persistent, or recurrent abscesses, the problem of antimicrobial therapy is certain to arise. In reaching a decision, one has to weigh the disadvantages of the drugs (see Table C-2, p. 161) against their potential benefit. There are no reports of local application of antimicrobials, but experience with other organisms suggests that this form of treatment is likely to be of limited value.

B. Pulmonary Lesions

When the disease is limited to a single lobe, and other features permit, resection has seemed to offer the best hope of effectuating a cure. Nine Japanese patients received resectional surgery, apparently without any notable complications.[394] However, in their patient, Nicholson and Sevier[266] observed postresectional spread of the pulmonary disease, infection of the surgical wound, and costal osteomyelitis. Guest and his colleagues encountered less difficulty in their patient.[154]

If one may judge from the pathology described in pulmonary processes, it would be reasonable to regard the underlying disease—fibrosis, abscesses, suppuration—rather than the specific organism as the indication for resection. It would also seem essential to carry on the most effective antimicrobial regimen achievable for at least a week or two before resection and for perhaps a month subsequently.

C. Susceptibility of *M. fortuitum* and Antimicrobial Therapy

In 1957, Kushner *et al.*[213] reported that oxytetracycline at 10 μg/ml inhibited 8 of 19 strains of *M. fortuitum*. In addition, they found 27 of 27 strains susceptible to isoniazid at 1 μg/ml and to tetracycline at 5 μg/ml. Other investigators[157,394] have presented findings at variance with this report, and Hawkins and McClean[163] have reported that all strains of rapidly growing organisms they tested were completely resistant to cycloserine at 50 μg/ml, a concentration far higher than one could achieve in clinical treatment. In addition, a Japanese group reported that 9 strains of *M. borstelense* (thought to be identical to *M. abscessus*) were completely resistant to all antimycobacterial drugs.

More recently, Clapper has reported strains that demonstrated susceptibility to kanamycin *in vitro*,[66] an observation that has received some
clinical support from the successful therapy of two very difficult problems.
In the report of Hand and Sanford,[159] an eight-year-old child developed an
abscess situated in the cauda equina; meningitis was also present. On the
basis of susceptibility *in vitro*, they treated with kanamycin daily, and to
this, for theoretical reasons, they added oxacillin. A complete cure followed. In the patient treated by Chusid *et al.*,[62] a paraspinal abscess had
developed and had extended to involve one pleural cavity, from the fluid of
which the organism was isolated. Pleural fluid was withdrawn, the abscess
was drained surgically, and the patient received a regimen of kanamycin,
ethambutol, isoniazid, and rifampin.

From this discussion, it is obvious that a decision to use drugs in the
treatment of a process caused by organisms such as *M. fortuitum* or *M.
abscessus* must hinge on the specific condition encountered. As is
suggested by the report of Awe *et al.*,[10] a period of observation before any
decision is reached is reasonable, unless there is some potentially lethal
process such as meningitis. In the case of pulmonary disease, the decisive
factor must be evidence of progression. Clearly, any regimen undertaken
should contain kanamycin on a daily basis. The addition of other drugs is
necessarily dependent on *in vitro* tests for susceptibility. If these tests
demonstrate total resistance to achievable concentrations, administration of
oxacillin and possibly of rifampin may provide increased antibiotic effect,
at least in theory.

13

Mycobacterium ulcerans

In 1948, MacCallum and associates[233] described a newly identified mycobacterial disease of the skin. It was marked by extensive undermining ulceration, and tissues revealed many acid-fast organisms. So far as they knew, the disease was limited to an area around Bairnsdale, on the southeast coast of Australia, almost directly east of Melbourne.

I. BACTERIOLOGY

The original description stated that the organism was definitely acid-fast, grew only between 30° and 35°, and produced small, domed colonies that later became lemon- or mustard-yellow on Petragnani's medium. Subsequently, Clancey isolated from similar dermal lesions of Ugandans a mycobacterium that he regarded as a new species (*Mycobacterium buruli*).[64] Like the Australian organism, the African organism displayed optimum growth at 32°–33° and formed low, convex colonies that were difficult to pick and that did not disperse well. In color, they were pale cream to light yellow, and they resembled *M. ulcerans* in negative oxidase and peroxidase reactions and in reducing nitrate rather slowly. They differed in that they produced a strongly positive neutral red reaction and also in their resistance to salicylate. In spite of these differences, the two organisms are now regarded as identical, as indicated by the work of Schröder,[331] whose study of all available strains led him to the conclusion that *M. buruli* is not a distinct species.

145

II. PATHOLOGY AND PATHOGENESIS

In their original report, the authors stated that the changes in the skin did not resemble tuberculosis. Dodge, in a more extensive description of lesions observed in Uganda,[98] reported that tissues revealed great numbers of organisms, which appeared extracellularly and at the spreading margin of the ulcer. The inflammatory reaction consisted of a narrow zone of polymorphonuclears, succeeded by an infiltration of lymphocytes, plasma cells, histiocytes, and large mononuclears. No caseation and only rare granulomas were found. The base of the ulcer displayed necrosis, probably the result of secondary infection. Occasional small areas of calcification were encountered, even though caseating necrosis was not present.

The pathological description provided by Connor and Lunn[72] agreed in its principal points with that of Dodge. They noted also an absence of reactive hyperemia at the margin of necrosis. Here and there, they also found lipid and foreign-body granulomas, with a rare noncaseating tuberculoid granuloma. These granulomas were conspicuous chiefly when the lesion had reached "the organizing stage."

In experimental studies of pathogenesis, Dodge found that organisms injected in the footpads of mice produced a slowly developing induration followed by ulceration. In males, scrotal swelling was a rather constant feature. Tolhurst *et al.* reported that after injection, lesions were discernible after 3–4 weeks and persisted for as long as 32 weeks. In young calves, subcutaneous injection of organisms produced ulcers similar to the human disease, and injected animals developed positive tuberculin tests.[382] Injection of *M. ulcerans* into the footpad of mice may also result in characteristic lesions of the tails.[233]

As explanation of the rapid, undermining necrosis, Connor and Lunn[72] argued that the essential lesion consisted of necrotizing panniculitis and postulated that the organism might release some fibrinolytic substance. Subsequently, with Krieg and Hochmeyer, Connor was able to confirm this supposition by the demonstration of a soluble substance in the culture filtrate that produced lesions in animals quite similar to those that followed injection of the organism.[203]

In the view of all these investigators, human infection probably occurs through inoculation or through previously existing abrasions or other superficial wounds. The infection remains confined to the skin and the immediately subjacent tissue, on account of the organism's requirement of lower temperatures for growth.

III. EPIDEMIOLOGY

A. Geographic Distribution

According to Reid, the disease has been encountered, usually in isolated pockets, in Australia, Africa, Papua, and Mexico.[302] Most of the African cases have been identified in the Buruli region of Uganda,[65] in Ubuje,[307] and in the Congo along its border with Uganda.[72] Proximity to rivers[72,302] or swampy areas[307] appears as a local feature within the more general distribution. One example of the disease, in a Nigerian immigrant, has been encountered in New York.[228]

B. Age

In the Port Moresby cases, the youngest patient was only 3 weeks old, while the oldest was 32 years.[302] Among Congolese, the average age was 12.5 years, while nearly all Ugandans were less than 30 years old.[72] Half of Dodge's patients were between 5 and 14 years of age.[98]

C. Sex

Only in the Port Moresby collection does mention of distribution occur: in that series of patients, males predominated over females 2:1.

D. Other Factors

Clancey and his associates described a familial distribution of disease,[65] while Revill and Barker[307] observed that the season of the year influenced the appearance of new cases. The irregular distribution by the month led them to suspect that the onset of a wetter period caused the growth of new grass, and they suspected that the organisms might have a natural distribution on these fresh sprouts. While some kind of environmental source of these organisms seems almost certain, no studies have demonstrated the existence of the organism outside the human body. Obviously water, soil, vegetation, and possibly even such things as sleeping mats may have to be examined before the exact pathway of infection can be established.

IV. CLINICAL FEATURES

Among both Buruli and Papuans, lesions usually appeared on the extensor surfaces of the extremities,[98,302] and 90% of the lesions reported from Uganda were situated on the legs or arms.[72] One infection reported from Mexico involved the palm of the hand.[217]

In most cases, the infection begins as a single subcutaneous nodular lesion.[98] The area gradually breaks down to form a single ulcer, and then spreading takes place beneath the skin, with extensive undermining. Pain is a very minor feature.[65] Connor and Lunn observed one individual in whom the original subcutaneous nodule did not ulcerate and another in which *M. ulcerans* produced a diffuse thickening and crusting.[72] Penetration of an ulcer of the leg into the cortex of the tibia has been observed once,[72] and Reid once encountered periostitis and twice encountered the destruction of muscle by a deepening ulceration.[302]

V. TREATMENT

For the concomitant secondary infection, Clancey *et al.* employed tetracycline.[65] After the tissues developed clean granulations, they resorted to debridement and extensive grafting. Reid[302] relied especially on the application of heat, followed by radical excision and grafts. In three cases in which recurrent ulceration occurred, Clancey and his associates used a streptomycin–isoniazid regimen with what appeared to be good results.[65] The palmar infection healed after eight months of administration of oxytetracycline and di-amino diphenylsulfone (a compound used in the treatment of leprosy.)

PART VI

APPENDIX

Appendix A

The Mycobacteria in Clinical Specialties

This short outline is meant to provide a general view of the specific infections that a specialist may encounter. More complete accounts of the processes are found in the chapters dealing with individual organisms. It should be remembered that the atypical mycobacteria constitute only one group of a large number of different organisms that produce granulomatous reactions. Most of the manifestations described may result from infection with tuberculosis or with almost any pathogenic fungus. The second imperative admonition is that many of these processes may occur in an altered host and that simple histological study may fail to identify processes. Study of biopsied material should include special stains for fungi and mycobacteria, even though the pathologist may report absence of granulomatous disease.

I. DERMATOLOGY

A. Hyperimmune Reactions

Erythema nodosum, erythema induratum, and erythema multiforme have all been observed in cases of disseminated infections of *M. kansasii*. In local or limited infections, dermatological lesions either have not appeared or have attracted no interest.

With disseminated infection caused by *M. intracellulare,* only erythema nodosum has been observed.

Macular lesions of the trunk have appeared in widespread infections due to either of these organisms, but since no biopsies were performed, it is not known if these lesions represented local cutaneous deposits of organisms or resulted from allergic response to some of the circulating antigens.

Mycobacterium intracellulare and *M. kansasii* account for most cases of disseminated mycobacteriosis, and the lack of reported dermatological lesions as a result of other organisms should not lead to the assumption that in a rare instance, lesions of the skin may not appear. It should also be considered that disseminated mycobacteriosis almost always occurs in a host with other disease that may seriously impair his immunity or in an individual whose immunity has been much impaired by therapy, as with corticosteroids.

B. Lesions Resulting from Organisms Directly

Nodular cutaneous and subcutaneous lesions of the scalp occurred in a young child with widely disseminated infection with *M. intracellulare.* The macular lesions mentioned above may belong to this group as well. It would be anticipated that occasionally other mycobacteria might produce the same types of disease.

C. Inoculation

Characteristic of this group of diseases are those that result from *M. marinum* and *M. ulcerans.* Both organisms require culture at lower temperatures and may be missed unless the laboratory receives notice that such an organism is suspected.

Mycobacterium marinum is widely distributed. In children, outbreaks may occur in epidemic form as a result of infection of the water of a swimming pool. Sporadic cases develop in connection with the cleaning of aquariums, with fishing, and with similar activities that involve contact with fish or their surroundings. The lesion usually consists of a violaceous nodule or a cluster of nodules. Evolution is slow and may result either in small apical ulcers or in crusting and wartlike lesions. Occasionally, sporotrichoid lesions may extend upward along an extremity. Most frequently, lymph nodes are not involved in the process.

Mycobacterium ulcerans has a much more limited distribution, and has been reported chiefly from Uganda and Papua. At a time when migration is frequent, immigrants from endemic areas may manifest the infection only after their arrival. The initial lesion is usually a nodule. In the course of four to six weeks, this lesion breaks down to form an ulcer that extends down to subcutaneous tissue. Undermining is a very striking feature, and ulceration may extend widely. Sometimes, however, ulceration is incomplete and the manifestation consists of extensive crusted, hyperkeratotic lesions.

Primary inoculation, similar to the primary inoculation of tuberculosis, occurs occasionally. Almost any of the more pathogenic mycobacteria may be the agent. Usually, the site is on the hand, where the lesion consists of a dull reddish papule that may slowly ulcerate. Extension is upward along the draining lymphatics and may resemble sporotrichosis, as is true of an infection with *M. kansasii*. Serpiginous and plaquelike lesions have resulted from similar inoculation of *M. intracellulare*. Infection with organisms that grow at 37° is likely to extend to the draining node.

II. ORTHOPEDIC SURGERY

Isolated infections of tendon sheaths have resulted from infection with *M. kansasii, M. intracellulare,* and *M. scrofulaceum.* These have characteristically developed slowly and with relatively little pain. Chronicity is characteristic of these infections, which relapse if removal is incomplete. Draining sinuses have not been reported. There is no clear evidence of a site of inoculation.

Osteomyelitis has occurred as a phase of disseminated disease, most commonly in young individuals with *M. intracellulare* infections. Much less commonly, these various types of infection have been associated with *M. scrofulaceum* and *M. abscessus.* Involvement has included both flat and long bones and has even affected the small bones of the hands and feet. Sometimes the disease is limited to a single bone, where it presents the appearance of a cyst. Draining sinuses and perforation into adjacent joint spaces have been reported. Characteristic disease of the vertebral column, similar to Pott's disease caused by *M. tuberculosis,* has not been encountered, nor has disease of the hip joint.

Isolated infection of bursae has been produced by *M. scrofulaceum, M. kansasii,* and *M. szulgai.*

Deep abscesses, without obvious connection to bone or to any underlying structure, have resulted from injections of many kinds of substances or have been associated with penetrating wounds. Practically all of these lesions have resulted from *M. abscessus.*

III. GENITOURINARY INFECTIONS

The most common cause of infection of the urinary tract has been *M. intracellulare.* Lesions have varied from hematuria without demonstrable pyelographic abnormality to destruction of a kidney.

Perirenal abscess seems to occur more commonly than in tuberculous infection. Apparently, only in one case has the infection resulted in a small, contracted bladder, and *M. intracellulare* so far has not been reported as involving other parts of the system.

Mycobacterium kansasii has been identified once as the etiological agent of epididymitis and once as a cause of both epididymitis and orchitis.

Caution: On several occasions, *M. intracellulare* and a very similar organism, *M. xenopi,* have been cultured from urine in the absence of any demonstrable disease. The frequency with which organisms can be cultured and the numbers of colonies probably constitute the best guide as to further investigation: in most situations in which the infection possesses clinical importance, cultures prove positive repeatedly and colonies are numerous.

IV. HEMATOLOGY

The most severe and extensive hematogenous infections with atypical mycobacteria, particularly *M. kansasii* or *M. intracellulare,* have occurred in individuals with hematological disorders. These have included pancytopenia, chronic granulocytic leukemia, or leukopenias of unknown cause. In cases with leukopenia or pancytopenia, it has often been uncertain if the organism produced the condition or the hematological disorder preceded the infection. In most instances, authors have speculated that infection followed upon the hematopoietic disorder.

Aspirated marrow has sometimes revealed granulomas, but often they are very poor formed and in some cases apparently have not been identified at all. In these instances, acid-fast stains and subsequently cultures have revealed the presence of mycobacteria. These studies should never be omitted in the investigation of unexplained fever in an individual whose primary problem is leukopenia or pancytopenia or in a patient who has developed these conditions as a result of treatment.

Appendix B

Alternate Classifications of Atypical Mycobacteria

The classification of Runyon did not receive total support, and several other arrangements of atypical mycobacteria have been suggested. In fairness, it is important to note that Runyon proposed his system very early in the period of renewed interest in atypical mycobacteria and that his classification was designed at a time when only few of the current tests had been established. Moreover, the intent was to produce a readily recognizable framework, suitable for use in less sophisticated laboratories.

In 1962, Collins[70] undertook to reorder mycobacteria with special reference to those isolated from human sources. His assemblages of organisms in four groups excluded *M. avium,* and he also set apart as not properly belonging to any of the assemblies *M. ulcerans, M. balnei, M. smegmatis,* and *M. phlei.* The four assemblies in themselves correspond to such tests as resistance to thiosemicarbazone, growth on simple media, and growth at 44°. Collins regarded organisms in his Assembly D as probably being partially separable from *M. fortuitum.* It is obvious that the exclusion of so many organisms renders this classification rather awkward to manage, although reliable bacteriological features underlie the schema.

At about the same time as Collins, Marks and Richards also undertook to arrange atypical mycobacteria in a pattern more inclusive than Collins's and more detailed than Runyon's. The essence of the system was consideration of a larger number of characteristics,[243] especially with respect to organisms of Runyon's Group III, which all investigators recognized as highly heterogeneous. The system offered by Marks and Richards,[243] in a somewhat simplified version, follows.

Group I was essentially the same as Runyon's, with *M. kansasii* the type strain or species.

Group II was restricted to *M. scrofulaceum* in an effort to exclude the usually nonpathogenic *M. aquae*.

Group III consisted of organisms that grew best at 42° but also fairly well at 45°. Pigmentation was very light and variable, and mycobacteria of this type were found to be sensitive to INH but resistant to thiosemicarbazone.

Group IV resembled Group III, except that growth was best at 45°. These organisms closely resembled *M. avium* and were resistant to all the usual antimycobacterial drugs except cycloserine.

Group V were dysgonic nonchromogenic organisms that could not tolerate temperature above 37°. They proved to be resistant to thiosemicarbazone.

Group VI produced eugonic growth in two to six days at 37° and were nonchromogenic, but unlike the organisms of Groups III, IV, and V, they were strongly catalase-positive.

Group VII resembled Group VI, except that growth was butyrous and required 25°.

Groups IV, V and VI were pathogenic, while Groups III and VII were not. The authors acknowledged that these subdivisions of nonchromogenic organisms lacked definition, but their studies and classifications served to set aside for special interest and study a group of organisms from which several species would ultimately be differentiated.

In 1964, Wayne[417] published a critique of various efforts at taxonomy. He regarded Runyon's Group I as well established but Groups II and III as very heterogeneous. He was particularly concerned that nearly all efforts at systematization had tended to regard *M. tuberculosis* as the organism against which all others were to be compared and prophetically wrote: "*M. tuberculosis* is not the sun, but rather one of the planets," and not a central one; it occupies "a very peripheral position, where its sharply limited distribution in nature suggests it belongs."

Just how peripheral in the genus of the mycobacteria *M. tuberculosis* is became clear only as Adansonian analysis came to be applied to a larger

number of traits. On the basis of studies of some 97 features of mycobacteria, Tsukamura and Mizuno[392] proposed in 1968 that the mycobacteria
might be divided into two major subgenera and that the relationships
among the members of the genus might be expressed by means of a den-
drogram (Figure B-1, modified from the original by omission of a scale of
similarity).

This ordering reflects the results of numerous enzymatic and biochemical tests and does not necessarily correspond with antigenic similarity.
However, the placement of *M. kansasii* near *M. tuberculosis* does agree
with similar placement on the basis of antigenic structure. The apposition
of *M. scrofulaceum* to the *avium–intracellulare* organisms likewise dis-
plays a relationship suggested by other modes of approach. Obviously,
classification of the mycobacteria remains fluid.

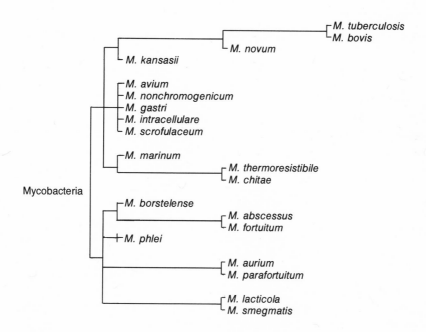

Figure B-1. Modified from Figure 2, Tsukamura and Mizuno, *Jap. J. Microbiol. 12:* 371–
384 (1968).

Appendix C

Drugs: Dosages, Toxicities, and Combinations

TABLE C-2
Dosages

Drug	Symbol	Dose	Frequency
Rifampin	RMP	600 mg/day	Single dose
Isoniazid[a]	INH	300 mg/day	t.i.d.
Ethambutol[b]	EMB	15 mg/kg/day	Single dose
p-Aminosalicylic acid	PAS	200 mg/kg/day	t.i.d.
Streptomycin[c]	SM	1.0 g	Daily or 2–3 times/week
Capreomycin	CM	1.0 g	As for SM
Kanamycin	KM	1.0 g	As for SM
Viomycin	VM	1.09 g	As for SM
Ethionamide	ETH	600 mg/day	b.i.d.
Cycloserine	CS	500 mg/day	b.i.d.
Pyrazinamide	PZA	1.5 g/day	t.i.d.
Erythromycin		1.0 g/day	q.i.d.
Sulfonamides		4.0 g/day	q.i.d.

[a]Pediatricians have followed the custom of using very much higher doses of INH, up to 12–15 mg/kg/day. The rationale offered is dubious, in that repeated studies have failed to demonstrate the advantage of high over low dose (4–5 mg/kg) and toxicity increases in proportion to dose. Pyridoxine 25–50 mg/day should always be used with higher doses.
[b]Many clinicians prefer to start EMB at 25 mg/kg and reduce to 15 mg/kg after one or two months. There appears to be no advantage in the higher dose and the risk of damage to the optic nerve is increased.
[c]It is usual to discontinue SM after four to six months, but if it is one of the more effective substances in a regimen, it may be continued, especially on a twice-weekly basis, for as much as two years. The same duration applies to KM and CM, provided there is no important renal or other toxicity.

TABLE C-2
Toxicities[a]

INH	Hepatic, peripheral nerve
PAS	Gastrointestinal
RMP	Renal (especially with interrupted doses)
EMB	Optic neuritis
ETH	Gastrointestinal; neural; thyroid
SM	8th nerve
CM	8th nerve; renal
KM	8th nerve; renal
CS	Central nervous system; confusion.
PZA	Hepatic (rare at 1.5 g daily)

[a]It should be understood that all of these substances may result in rashes, serum-sickness syndrome, and similar allergic disorders. Idiosyncratic responses, such as depression of bone marrow, are uncommon.

TABLE C-3
Probable Effective Regimens[a]

Group I	M. kansasii	3-drug regimen preferred: INH or RMP–SM–EMB.
	M. marinum	RMP–EMB; additional SM or ETH; Sulfamethoxazole? Trimethoprim?
Group II	M. scrofulaceum	SM–RMP preferred; CS; PAS; ETH: KM?; Sulfadiazine? Erythromycin?
	M. gordonae	RMP–SM–EMB.
	M. szulgai	INH–RMP–SM; possibly EMB or ETH.
Group III	Avium-Battey complex	3–4 drug regimen essential: RMP–SM–EMB–CS.
	M. xenopi	Await specific susceptibility.
Group IV.	M. fortuitum	KM–RMP; EMB? Oxacillin?
	M. abscessus	Same.
Others	M. ulcerans	INH–SM.
	M. simiae	Await susceptibility.

[a]It should be understood and expected that as the number of drugs in the regimen increases, and particularly as it becomes necessary to resort to "second-line" substances, the probabilities of untoward effects and reactions increase disproportionately. For this reason, the following system of surveillance is recommended on all patients who receive three or more drugs.

TABLE C-4
Surveillance[a]

1. SGOT; alkaline phosphatase; bilirubin—monthly.
2. Visual acuity, if EMB is in the regimen—monthly.
3. Urinalysis and BUN—monthly.
4. Audiometry (for injectables)—monthly.
5. CBC—monthly.

[a]If reaction of a nonspecific type, such as rash, occurs, it is preferable to discontinue all medication and then to reintroduce one substance at a time, beginning with the ones least likely to produce trouble.

Glossary

In addition to the regularly used names of organisms throughout the text, at various times other names have been applied. Since revisions of nomenclature take place continuously, many references employ terms for organisms that have since been considered inappropriate. This list of names is intended to clarify references, especially some of the older ones. Even now, there is no universal agreement with respect to nomenclature.

Battey bacilli—a familiar term used in reference to members of Runyon's Group III. In most cases the implied organism is *M. intracellulare*.

Nonchromogens (also nonphotochromogens)—likewise an inclusive term sometimes intended to include all nonpigmented, slower-growing atypical mycobacteria. Synonymous in common usage with *Battey bacilli*.

Photochromogens—sometimes employed as a synonym for Runyon's Group I, but in common practice the term refers to *M. kansasii*, though of course there are other photochromogenic organisms.

Scotochromogens—an inclusive term that designates all members of Runyon's Group II.

Radish bacillus—a term familiarly employed to designate one of the *M. terrae* complex.

Timothy bacillus—familiar term for *M. phlei*.

In addition to these, many mycobacteria are referred to by names that have subsequently been superseded or discarded.

M. aquae—now known as *M. gordonae.*

M. balnei—preferred term, *M. marinum.*

M. borstelense—known variously at different times as *M. runyoni, M. chelonei, M. abscessus;* closely related to *M. fortuitum.*

M. brunense—now identified not as a species but as serotype Davis of *M. intracellulare.*

M. buruli—now shown to be identical with *M. ulcerans.*

M. chelonei—see *M. borstelense.*

M. gastri—apparently a species; formerly included with similar organisms in Wayne's J-group.

M. habana—established as identical to *M. simiae.*

M. laciflavum—applied at one time to *M. kansasii.*

M. nonchromogenicum—a nonpathogenic member of the *terrae* complex.

M. peregrinum—a variant strain of *M. fortuitum.*

M. runyoni—see *M. borstelense.*

M. triviale—a nonpathogenic organism speciated from other members of Wayne's V-group.

References

1. Abello, V. B., Riley, H. D., Jr., and Rubio, T., Atypical mycobacterial infections in children, *Scand. J. Infect. Dis. 3:*163–167 (1971).
2. Adams, R. M., Remington, J. S., Steinberg, J., and Seibert, J. S., Tropical fish aquariums. A source of *Mycobacterium marinum* infections resembling sporotrichosis, *J. Amer. Med. Assoc. 211:*457–461 (1970).
3. Ahn, C. H., Nash, D. R., and Hurst, G. A., Ventilatory defects in atypical mycobacteriosis, *Am. Rev. Respir. Dis. 113:*273–280 (1976).
4. Alshabkhoun, A., Chapman, P. T., White, M. F., and De Groat, A., A study of the double diffusion gel precipitation test in tuberculous patients with special reference to technical problems, *Am. Rev. Respir. Dis. 81:*704–708 (1960).
5. Andrejew, A., Phosphatase activity of mycobacteria, *Ann. Inst. Pasteur* (Paris) *115:*11–22 (1968).
6. Andrejew, A., and Gernez-Rieux, C., Éssais de différentiation des mycobactéries d'après la sensibilité de leur activité catalasique aux inhibiteurs, *Ann. Inst. Pasteur* (Paris) *103:*201–215 (1962).
7. Andrejew, A., Gernez-Rieux, C., and Tacquet, A., Activité peroxidasique des mycobactéries, *Ann. Inst. Pasteur* (Paris) *91:*586–589 (1956).
8. Arloing, S., Variations du bacille tuberculeux (specialement au point de vue de virulence), *6th Internatl. Cong. on Tuberc. 1:*Part 1, 68 (1908).
9. Atwell, R. J., and Pratt, P. C., Unclassified mycobacteria in the gastric contents of healthy personnel and patients of a tuberculosis hospital, *Am. Rev. Respir. Dis. 81:*888–892 (1960).
10. Awe, R. J. Gangadharam, P. R., and Jenkins, D. E., Clinical significance of *Mycobacterium fortuitum* in pulmonary disease, *Am. Rev. Respir. Dis. 108:* 1230–1234 (1973).
11. Bailey, R. K., Wyles, S., Dingley, M., Hesse, F., and Kent, G. W., The isolation of high catalase *Mycobacterium kansasii* from tap water, *Am. Rev. Respir. Dis. 101:*430–431 (1970).
12. Bailey, W. C., Brown, M., Buechner, H. A., Weill, H., Ichinose, H., and Ziskind, M., Silico-mycobacterial disease in sand-blasters, *Am. Rev. Respir. Dis. 110:*115–125 (1974).

167

13. Bannerjee, R., Hall, R., and Hughes, G. R. V., Pulmonary *Mycobacterium fortuitum* infection in association with achalasia of the oesophagus, *Br. J. Dis. Chest 64:*112–118 (1970).

14. Barbolini, G., Bisetti, A., and Pozzi, F., Esperienze sulla condizionata patogenecita dei micobatterie "anonimi" (ceppi M 4 and P1) nella cavia, *G. Mal. Infett. Parassit. 16:*659–665 (1964).

15. Barrow, G. L., and Hewitt, M., Skin infection with a Mycobacterium marinum from a *tropical fish tank. Ba. Med. J. 2:*505–506 (1971).

16. Bates, J. H., A study of pulmonary disease associated with mycobacteria other than *Mycobacterium tuberculosis:* Clinical characteristics, *Am. Rev. Respir. Dis. 96:*1151–1157 (1967).

17. Bates, R. D., and Chapman, J. S., Tuberculin test: some inherent limitations, *Tex. State J. Med. 60:*517–519 (1964).

18. Beaven, P. W., and Bayne-Jones, S., Mycobacterium (Sp?) Ryan strain isolated from pleural exudate, *J. Infect. Dis. 49:*399–419 (1931).

19. Beck, A., *Mycobacterium fortuitum* in abscesses of man, *J. Clin. Pathol.* (Lond.) *18:*307–313 (1965).

20. Beck, C. C., Ellis, D. J., Hoefer, J. A., Scott, R. M., and Stewart, J. M., Experiences and implication of an outbreak of swine tuberculosis in a university swine herd, *Proceedings of the 66th Annual Meeting of the U.S. Livestock Sanitary Association,* pp. 184–192 (1962).

21. Bel, F., Étude biochimique et sérologique de mycobactéries atypiques scoto-chromogènes isolées d'adénites. Thesis, presented to the Faculty of Sciences of the University of Lausanne, 1967.

22. Belcher, J. R., The pulmonary complications of dysphagia, *Thorax 4:* 44–56 (1949).

23. Benda, R., Stuhl, L., and Frey, N., Effets des radiations ionisantes de haute énergie sur le bacille de Koch et diverses mycobactéries atypiques, *Rev. Tuberc. Pneumol. 28:*997–1008 (1964).

24. Berman, D. T., Tervola, C. A., and Erdmann, A. A., Preliminary report of investigations of tuberculin sensitivity in Wisconsin cattle, *Proceedings of the 63rd Annual Meeting of the U.S. Livestock Sanitary Association,* pp. 197–204 (1959).

25. Bhadrakom, S., Thasnakorn, P., Prijyanonda, B., and Bovornkitti, S., Scotochromogenic acid-fast bacilli isolated from pleural aspirate, *J. Med. Assoc. Thailand 51:*33–38 (1968).

26. Bialkin, G., Pollak, A., and Weil, A. J., Pulmonary infection with *Mycobacterium kansasii, Am. J. Dis. Child. 101:*739–748 (1961).

27. Birn, K. J., Schaefer, W. B., Jenkins, P. A., Szulga, T., and Marks, J., Classification of *Mycobacterium avium* and related opportunistic mycobacteria met in England and Wales, *J. Hyg. 65:*575–589 (1967).

28. Bisetti, A., and Barbolini, G., Potere patogeno sperimentale di taluni ceppi micobatterie "anonimi" isolati nell'uomo in Emilia, *G. Mal. Infett. Parassit. 16:*646–657 (1964).

29. Bjerkedal, T., Mycobacterial infections in Norway: A preliminary note on determining their identity and frequency, *Am. J. Epidemiol. 85:*157–173 (1967).

30. Black, B. G., and Chapman, J. S., Cervical adenitis in children due to human and unclassified mycobacteria, *Pediatrics 33:*887–893 (1964).

31. Boisvert, H., *Mycobacterium xenopei* (Marks and Schwabacher, 1965), mycobactérie

scotochromogene, thermophile, dysgonique, éventuellement pathogène pour l'homme, *Ann. Inst. Pasteur* (Paris) *109:*447–453 (1965).

32. Bojalil, L. F., Cerbon, J., and Trujillo, A., Adansonian classification of mycobacteria, *J. Gen. Microbiol. 28:*333–346 (1962).

33. Bönicke, R., Über das Vorkommen von Acylamidasen in Mykobakterien. V. Die Identifizierung von "atypischen" Mykobakterien der photochromogenen Gruppe mit Hilfe der "Amid-Reihe," *Zentralbl. Bakteriol. Parasitenkd. Infectionskr. Hyg. Abt. 1 Orig. 179:*223–230 (1960).

34. Bönicke, R., Identification of mycobacteria by biochemical methods, *Bull. Int. Union Tuberc. 32:*13–68 (1962).

35. Borghans, J. G. A., and Stanford, J. L., *Mycobacterium chelonei* in abscesses after injection of diphtheria–tetanus–pertussis–polio vaccine, *Amer. Rev. Respir. Dis. 107:*1–8 (1973).

36. Boyd, G. L., and Craig, G., Etiology of cat-scratch fever, *J. Pediatr. 59:*313–317 (1961).

37. Brasher, C. A., personal communication, letter of Nov. 16, 1971.

38. Brock, J. M., Kennedy, C. B., and Clark, W. H., Jr., Cutaneous infection with atypical mycobacteria, *Arch. Dermatol. 82:*918–920 (1960).

39. Buhler, V. B., and Pollak, A., Human infection with atypical acid-fast organisms. Report of two cases with pathologic findings, *Am. J. Clin. Pathol. 23:*363–374 (1953).

40. Bullin, C. H., Tanner, E. I., and Collins, C. H., Isolation of *Mycobacterium xenopei* from water taps, *J. Hyg. 68:*97–100 (1970).

41. Burrell, R. G., Rheins, M., and Birkeland, J. M., Tuberculous antibodies demonstrated by agar diffusion. II. Further characterization of these antibodies and their distribution in human serum, *Am. Rev. Tuberc. Pulm. Dis. 74:*239–244 (1956).

42. Canetti, G., Some remarks on the diversity of criteria of resistance presently employed, *Bull. Int. Union Tuberc. 27:*224–228 (1957).

43. Canilang, B., and Armstrong, D., Subcutaneous abscesses due to *Mycobacterium fortuitum, Am. Rev. Respir. Dis. 97:*451–454 (1968).

44. Caplan, H., and Clayton, M., Carpal tunnel syndrome secondary to *Mycobacterium kansasii* infection, *J. Amer. Med. Assoc. 208:*1186–1188 (1969).

45. Carruthers, K. J. M., and Edwards, F. G. B., Atypical mycobacteria in Western Australia, *Am. Rev. Respir. Dis. 91:*887–895 (1965).

46. Cater, J. C., and Redmond, W. B., Isolation of and studies on bacteriophage active against mycobacteria, *Can. J. Microbiol. 7:*697–703 (1961).

47. Chapman, J. S., Atypical mycobacterial infections, *Med. Clin. North Am. 51:*503–517 (1971).

48. Chapman, J. S., The ecology of the atypical mycobacteria, *Arch. Environ. Health 22:*41–46 (1971).

49. Chapman, J. S., a review of early events in tubercle formation, *Acta Pathol. Microbiol. Scand. sect. A. Pathol., 803, Suppl. 233:*189–194 (1972).

50. Chapman, J. S., and Bernard, J. S., The tolerance of unclassified mycobacteria. 1. Limits of pH tolerance, *Am. Rev. Respir. Dis. 86:*582–583 (1962).

51. Chapman, J. S., Bernard, J. S., and Speight, M., Isolation of mycobacteria from raw milk, *Am. Rev. Respir. Dis. 91:*351–355 (1965).

52. Chapman, J. S., Clark, J., and Speight, M., Electrophoresis of antigens of atypical mycobacteria, *Am. Rev. Respir. Dis. 92, Part 2:*73–81 (1965).

53. Chapman, J. S., Dewlett, H. J., and Potts, W. E., Cutaneous reactions to unclassified mycobacterial antigens, *Am. Rev. Respir. Dis. 86:*547–552 (1962).

54. Chapman, J. S., Dyerly, M., and Spohn, S., Epidemiological notes on *Mycobacterium kansasii* disease, *Arch. Environ. Health 16:*673–678 (1968).

55. Chapman, J. S., and Guy, L. R., Scrofula caused by atypical mycobacteria, *Pediatrics 23:*323–331 (1959).

56. Chapman, J. S., and Speight, M., Further studies of mycobacterial antibodies in the sera of sarcoidosis patients, *Acta Med. Scand. 176, Suppl. 425:*61–66 (1964).

57. Chapman, J. S., and Speight, M., Isolation of atypical mycobacteria from pasteurized milk, *Am. Rev. Respir. Dis. 98:*1052–1054 (1968).

58. Chapman, J. S., and Speight, M., Tolerance of atypical mycobacteria: The effect of metal ions in various concentrations, *Am. Rev. Respir. Dis. 103:*372–376 (1971).

59. Chase, M. W., and Kawata, H., Multiple bacterial antigens in diagnostic tuberculins, *Dev. Biol. Stand. 29:*308–330 (1975).

60. Chicoine, L., Lapointe, N., Simoneau, R., and LaFleure, L., "Anonymous" mycobacterial infections causing disseminated osteomyelitis and skin lesions, *Can. Med. Assoc. J. 98:*1059–1062 (1968).

61. Christianson, L. C., and Dewlett, H. J., Pulmonary disease in adults associated with unclassified mycobacteria, *Am. J. Med. 29:*980–991 (1960).

62. Chusid, M. J., Parrillo, J. E., and Fauci, A. S., Chronic granulomatous disease. Diagnosis in a 27-year-old man with *Mycobacterium fortuitum, J. Amer. Med. Assoc. 233:*1295–1296 (1975).

63. Cianciulli, F. D., The radish bacillus (*Mycobacterium terrae*), saprophyte or pathogen? *Am. Rev. Respir. Dis. 109:*138–141 (1974).

64. Clancey, J. K., Mycobacterial skin ulcers in Uganda: Description of a new mycobacterium (*Mycobacterium buruli*), *J. Pathol. Bacteriol. 88:*175–187 (1964).

65. Clancey, J. K., Dodge, O. G., Lunn, H. F., and Odouri, M. L., Mycobacterial skin ulcers in Uganda, *Lancet 1961–2:*951–954.

66. Clapper, W. E., *Mycobacterium fortuitum* abscess at injection site (Letter), *J. Amer. Med. Assoc. 202:*550 (1967).

67. Clark, J., Thomson, D. S., and Wallace, A., Disseminated infection with *Mycobacterium avium:* Part II. Bacteriology and drug susceptibility, *Tubercle 49:*31–37 (1968).

68. Cohen, M. J., Matz, L. R., and Elphick, H. R., Infection of the soft tissues of the ankle by a Group II mycobacterium (scotochromogen), *Med. J. Aust. 1970–2:*679–681.

69. Cohen, S. S., personal communication.

70. Collins, C. H., The classification of "anonymous" acid-fast bacilli from human sources, *Tubercle 43:*292–298 (1962).

71. Comstock, G. W., A comparison of purified tuberculins in the Southeastern U.S.A., *Bull. W. H. O.* 23:683–688 (1960).

72. Connor, D. H., and Lunn, H. F., Buruli ulceration: A clinico-pathologic study of 38 Ugandans with *Mycobacterium ulcerans* ulceration, *Arch. Pathol. 81:*183–199 (1966).

73. Cooper, A. R., and Martin, R. S., Pulmonary *Mycobacterium scrofulaceum* in a child, *Pediatrics 49:*118–123 (1972).

74. Corpe, R. F., Clinical aspects, medical and surgical, in the management of Battey-type pulmonary disease, *Dis. Chest 45:*380–382 (1964).

75. Corpe, R. F., Runyon, E. H., and Lester, W., Status of disease due to unclassified mycobacteria: A statement of the subcommittee on unclassified mycobacteria of the Committee on Therapy, *Am. Rev. Respir. Dis. 87:*459–461 (1963).

76. Corpe, R. F., Smith, C. E., and Stergus, I., Death due to *Mycobacterium fortuitum*, *J. Amer. Med. Assoc. 177:*262–263 (1961).

77. Corpe, R. F., and Stergus, I., Is histopathology of nonphotochromogenic mycobacterial infection distinguishable from that caused by *Mycobacterium tuberculosis? Am. Rev. Respir. Dis. 87:*289–291 (1963).

78. Cott, R. E., Carter, D. M., and Sall, T., Cutaneous disease caused by atypical mycobacteria, *Arch. Dermatol. 95:*259–268 (1967).

79. Courmont, P., and Potet, M., Les bacilles acido-résistants du beurre, du lait, et de la nature, comparés au bacille de Koch, *Arch. Med. Exp. 15:*83–128 (1903).

80. Cowie, D. M., A preliminary report on acid-resisting bacilli with special reference to their occurrence in lower animals, *J. Exp. Med. 5:*205–214 (1900).

81. Crawford, A. B., Studies in avian tuberculosis. 4. The possible role of the avian tubercle bacillus in infection in man, *Am. Rev. Tuberc. 37:*594–597 (1938).

82. Crompton, G. K., Schonell, M. E., and Wallace, A., Disseminated infection with *Mycobacterium avium:* Part III. Sensitivity to avian tuberculin among contacts, *Tubercle 49:*38–41 (1968).

83. Crowle, A. J., and Hu, C. C., Specificity of inhibition by antiserum of the development of immediate and delayed hypersensitivities in mice, *Proc. Soc. Exp. Biol. Med. 127:*190–193 (1968).

84. Cuttino, J. T., and McCabe, A. M., Pure granulomatous nocardiosis: A new fungus disease distinguished by intracellular parasitism. A description of a new disease in man due to a hitherto undescribed organism, *Nocardia intracellulare* N. sp., including study of the biologic and pathologic properties of the species, *Am. J. Pathol. 25:*1–48 (1949).

85. Daniel, T. M., Observations on the antibody response of rabbits to mycobacterial antigens, *J. Immunol. 95:*100–108 (1965).

86. Daniel, T. M., and Todd, L. S., The species distribution of three concanavalin-A purified mycobacterial polysaccharides, *Am. Rev. Respir. Dis. 112:*361–364 (1975).

87. Daniel, T. M., and Wisnieski, J. J., The reaction of concanavalin-A with mycobacterial culture filtrates, *Am. Rev. Respir. Dis. 101:*762–764 (1970).

88. Danigelis, J. A., and Long, R. E., Anonymous mycobacterial osteomyelitis. A case report in a six-year-old child, *Radiology 93:*353–354 (1969).

89. David, H. L., Response of mycobacteria to ultraviolet light irradiation, *Am. Rev. Respir. Dis. 108:*1175–1185 (1973).

90. Davis, S. D., and Comstock, G. W., Mycobacterial cervical adenitis in children, *J. Pediatr. 58:*771–778 (1961).

91. Davis, S. D., Kirby, W. M. M., and Sherris, S. C., Disseminated osteomyelitis due to "Battey" mycobacteria, *Am. Rev. Respir. Dis. 93:*269–274 (1966).

92. Dechairo, D. C., Kittredge, D., Meyers, A., and Corrales, J., Septic arthritis due to *Mycobacterium triviale, Am. Rev. Respir. Dis. 108:*1224–1226 (1973).

93. Decroix, G., Bresland, P., and Kourilsky, R., Titrage d'un anticorps polysaccharidique tuberculeux dans le sérum de malades atteints de syndromes ganglio-pulmonaires avec réactions tuberculiniques négatives, *J. Franc. Med. Thor. 9:*638–651 (1955).

94. D'Esopo, N. D., Preliminary report of study of disease due to mycobacteria other than *M. tuberculosis, Transactions of the 24th Research Conference in Pulmonary Disease,* pp. 70–74 (1965).

95. Diaz, G. A., and Wayne, L. G., Isolation and characterization of catalase produced by *Mycobacterium tuberculosis, Am. Rev. Respir. Dis. 110:*312–319 (1974).

96. Dickey, R. F., Sporotrichoid mycobacteriosis caused by *M. marinum (balnei), Arch. Dermatol. 98:*385–391 (1968).

97. Dieterlen (no initials given), Zur Frage der im Auswurf Lungenkranker vorkommenden Tuberkelbazillen, *Dtsch. Med. Wochenschr. 36:*207–209 (1910).

98. Dodge, O. G., Mycobacterial skin ulcers in Uganda: Histopathological and experimental aspects, *J. Pathol. Bacteriol. 88:*169–184 (1964).

99. Donovan, W. N., Krasnow, I., Donowho, E. M., Jr., and Johanson, W. G., Jr., *Mycobacterium simiae, Am. Rev. Respir. Dis. 113, No. 4, Part 2:*55 (abst.) (1976).

100. Doyle, W. M., Evander, L. C., and Gruft, H., Pulmonary disease caused by *Mycobacterium xenopei, Am. Rev. Respir. Dis. 97:*912–922 (1968).

101. Dragsted, I., Avian tuberculosis in man. *Lancet 1949 2:*103–105.

102. Dubos, R. J., and Middlebrook, G., Cytochemical reactions of virulent tubercle bacilli, *Am. Rev. Tuberc. 58:*698–699 (1948).

103. Duvall, C. W., Studies in atypical forms of tubercle bacilli isolated directly from the human tissues in cases of primary cervical adenitis, *J. Exp. Med. 9:*403–429 (1908).

104. Edwards, L. B., Hopwood, L., Affronti, L., and Palmer, C. E., Sensitivity profiles of mycobacterial infections, *Bull. Int. Union Tuberc. 32:*373–384 (1962).

105. Edwards, L. B., and Krohn, E. F., Skin sensitivity to antigens made from various acid-fast bacteria, *Am. J. Hyg. 66:*253–273 (1957).

106. Edwards, L. B., and Palmer, C. E., Epidemiological studies of tuberculin sensitivity. I. Preliminary results with purified protein derivatives prepared from atypical acid-fast organisms, *Am. J. Hyg. 68:*213–229 (1958).

107. Edwards, L. B., and Palmer, C. E., Isolation of "atypical" mycobacteria from healthy persons, *Am. Rev. Respir. Dis. 80:*747–749 (1959).

108. Elston, H. R., and Duffy, C. P., *Mycobacterium xenopi* and mycobacteriosis. A clinical and bacteriologic report, *Am. Rev. Respir. Dis. 108:*944–949 (1973).

109. Elston, H. R., Parrillo, O. J., Meiberger, M., and Kleitsch, P., Pulmonary mycobacteriosis. Report of seven cases. *Arch. Intern. Med. 113:*365–372 (1964).

110. Engbaek, H. C., Three cases in the same family of fatal infection with *M. avium, Acta Tuberc. Scand. 45:*105–117 (1964).

111. Engbaek, H. C., Friis, T., and Ohlsen, A. S., A case of lung disease caused by an atypical acid-fast organism, *Acta Tuberc. Scand. 34:*145–162 (1957).

112. Engbaek, H. C., Vergman, B., Baess, I., and Weis Bentzon, M., *Mycobacterium avium,*. A bacteriological and epidemiological study of *M. avium* isolated from animals and man in Denmark. Part 1. Strains isolated from animals. *Acta Pathol Microbiol. Scand. 72:*277–294 (1968).

113. Engbaek, H. C., Vergman, B., Baess, I., and Weis Bentzon, M., *Mycobacterium avium.* A bacteriological and epidemiological study of *M. avium* isolated from animals and man in Denmark. Part 2. Strains isolated from man, *Acta Pathol. Microbiol. Scand. 72:*295–312 (1968).

114. Engbaek, H. C., Vergman, B., Baess, I., and Will, D. W., *M. xenopi.* A bacteriological study of *M. xenopi,* including case reports of Danish patients, *Acta Pathol. Microbiol. Scand. 69:*576–594 (1967).

115. Engstrom, P. F., Dewey, G. C., and Barrett, O., Disseminated *Mycobacterium kansasii* infection. Successful treatment of a patient with pancytopenia, *Am. J. Med. 52:*533–537 (1972).

116. Faber, D. R., Lasky, I. I., and Goodwin, W. E., Idiopathic unilateral renal hematuria

associated with atypical acid-fast bacillus: Battey type. Cured by partial nephrectomy, *J. Urol. 93:*435–439 (1965).

117. Falk, G. A., Hadley, S. J., Sharkey, F. E., Liss, M., and Muschenheim, C., *Mycobacterium avium* infections in man, *Am. J. Med. 54:*801–810 (1973).

118. Feinberg, K. A., and Schneierson, S. S., Disseminated infection by *Mycobacterium fortuitum, J. Mt. Sinai Hosp. 36:*375–379 (1969).

119. Feldman, R. A., and Hershfield, E., Mycobacterial skin infection by an unidentified species. A report of 29 patients. *Ann. Intern. Med. 80:*445–452 (1974).

120. Feldman, W. H., and Auerbach, O., Histopathology of granulomatous pulmonary lesions associated with Battey-type mycobacteria, *Transactions of the 22nd Research Conference in Pulmonary Disease,* pp. 239–242 (1963).

121. Feldman, W. H., Davies, R., Moses, H. E., and Andberg, W., An unusual mycobacterium isolated from the sputum of a man suffering from pulmonary disease of long duration, *Am. Rev. Tuberc. 48:*82–93 (1943).

122. Feldman, W. H., Hutchinson, D. W., Schwarting, V. M., and Karlson, A. G., Juvenile tuberculous infection, probably of avian type, *Am. J. Pathol. 25:*1183–1196 (1949).

123. Fischer, D. A., Lester, W., and Schaefer, W. B., Infections with atypical mycobacteria. Five years' experience at the National Jewish Hospital, *Am. Rev. Respir. Dis. 98:*29–34 (1968).

124. Fisher, S., An epidemiological survey of mycobacterial disease in New South Wales, 1965–1969, *Med. J. Aust. 1971–1:*1047–1053.

125. Flowers, D. J., Human infection with *Mycobacterium marinum* after a dolphin bite, *J. Clin. Pathol. 23:*475–477 (1970).

126. Francis, P. B., Jay, S. J., and Johanson, W. G., Jr., The course of untreated *M. kansasii* disease, *Am. Rev. Respir. Dis. 111:*477–488 (1975).

127. Fraser, D. W., Buxton, A. E., Naji, A., Barker, C. F., Rudnick, M., and Weinstein, A. J., Disseminated *Mycobacterium kansasii* infection presenting as a cellulitis in a recipient of a renal homograft, *Am. Rev. Respir. Dis. 112:*125–130 (1975).

128. Freeman, G., Unusual mycobacterial infections, *Am. Rev. Tuberc. 38:*612–623 (1938).

129. Gacad, G., and Massaro, D., Pulmonary fibrosis and Group IV mycobacteria infection of the lung in ankylosing spondylitis, *Am. Rev. Respir. Dis. 109:*274–278 (1974).

130. Gangadharam, P. R., and Droubi, A. J., Susceptibility of mycobacteria to *p*-nitrobenzoic acid in relation to their niacin production, *Am. Rev. Respir. Dis., 108:*143–146 (1973).

131. Gangadharam, P. R., and Hsu, K. H. K., *Mycobacterium abscessus* infection in a puncture wound, *Am. Rev. Respir. Dis. 106:*275–277 (1972).

132. Garcia, O. P., and Santos, C., Notes on a Loeffler-like syndrome in guinea-pigs inoculated with atypical acid-fast bacilli, *Bull. Quezon Inst. 1959:*49–56.

133. Gernez-Rieux, C., and Tacquet, A., Les infections humaines a mycobactéries ''atypiques'' au cours de pneumoconioses. Étude clinique et expérimentale. *Bull. Int. Union Tuberc. 29:*330–342 (1959).

134. Gernez-Rieux, C., Tacquet, A., and Macquet, V., Les affections pulmonaires dues aux mycobactéries atypiques, *Pathol. Biol. 8:*1667–1681 (1960).

135. Gibson, J. B., Infection of the lungs by saprophytic mycobacteria in achalasia of the cardia, with report of a fatal case showing lipoid pneumonia due to milk, *J. Pathol. Bacteriol. 65:*239–251 (1953).

136. Gilkerson, S. W., Moss, M., and Cuthrell, F., Microculture morphology of mycobacteria, *J. Bacteriol. 91*:1652–1654 (1966).

137. Girard, D. E., Bagby, C. C., Jr., and Walsh, J. R., Destructive polyarthritis due to *Mycobacterium kansasii, Arthritis Rheum. 16*:665–669 (1973).

138. Godwin, M. C., Infection of knee joint by *Mycobacterium kansasii, J. Amer. Med. Assoc. 194*:88–89 (1965).

139. Goldman, K. P., Treatment of unclassified mycobacterial infection of the lungs, *Thorax 23*:94–99 (1968).

140. Gonzales, E. P., Crosby, R. M. N., and Walker, S. H., *Mycobacterium aquae* infection in a hydrocephalic child, *Pediatrics 48*:974–977 (1971).

141. Gordon, R. E., The classification of acid-fast bacteria, *J. Bacteriol. 34*:617–630 (1937).

142. Goslee, S., and Wolinsky, M., Water as a source of potentially pathogenic mycobacteria, *Am. Rev. Respir. Dis. 113*:287–292 (1976).

143. Graybill, J. R., Silva, J., Fraser, D. W., Lordon, R., and Rogers, E., Disseminated mycobacteriosis due to *Mycobacterium abscessus* in two recipients of renal homografts, *Am. Rev. Respir. Dis. 109*:4–10 (1974).

144. Green, H. H., *in* Discussion on tuberculins in human and veterinary medicine, *Proc. R. Soc. Med. 44*:1045–1050 (1951).

145. Grigelova, R., Turzova, M., Dornetzhuber, V., and Urbancik, R., A contribution to the problem of lymphatic system diseases provoked in children by *Mycobacterium avium, Scand. J. Respir. Dis. 48*:71–75 (1967).

146. Grillo-Lopez, A. J., Rivera, E., Castillo-Staab, M., and Maldonado, N., Disseminated *M. kansasii* infection in a patient with chronic granulocytic leukemia, *Cancer 28*:476–481 (1971).

147. Gross, W., Hawkins, J. E., and Murphy, D. B., *Mycobacterium xenopi* in clinical specimens. Water as a source of contamination (abst.), *Am. Rev. Respir. Dis. 113, No. 4, Part 2*:78 (1976).

148. Gruft, H., Strains of *Mycobacterium kansasii* with weak catalase activity, *Am. Rev. Respir. Dis. 106*:119–120 (1972).

149. Gruft, H., Blanchard, D., and Wheeler, J., Ocean waters a source of *Mycobacterium intracellulare* (abst.), *Am. Rev. Respir. Dis. 113, No. 4, Part 2*:60 (1976).

150. Gruft, H., and Gaafar, H. A., Multiple catalases of mycobacteria: Differences in molecular weight, *Am. Rev. Respir. Dis. 110*:320–323 (1974).

151. Gruft, H., and Henning, H. G., Pulmonary mycobacteriosis due to a rapidly growing acid-fast bacillus, *Mycobacterium chelonei, Am. Rev. Respir. Dis. 105*:618–620 (1972).

152. Gruhl, V. R., and Reese, M. H., Disseminated atypical mycobacterial disease presenting as "leukemia," *Am. J. Clin. Pathol. 55*:206–211 (1971).

153. Grzybowski, S., Brown, M. T., and Rowe, J. F., Significance of the tuberculin reaction, *Can. Med. Assoc. J. 100*:984–987 (1969).

154. Guest, J. L., Jr., Arean, V. M., and Brenner, H. A., Group IV mycobacterium infection occurring in association with mineral oil granuloma of the lungs, *Am. Rev. Respir. Dis. 95*:656–662 (1967).

155. Gunnel, J. J., and Bates, J. H., Characterization and mycobacteriophage typing of *Mycobacterium xenopi, Am. Rev. Respir. Dis. 105*:388–392 (1972).

156. Gursel, A., *et al.* (sic), Preliminary study of acid-fast bacilli isolated from samples of

earth in Ankara, *Tuberk. Toraks. 6:*483–489 (1970). Abst. in *Am. Rev. Respir. Dis. 104:*309 (1971).

157. Guy, L. R., and Chapman, J. S., Susceptibility *in vitro* of unclassified mycobacteria to commonly used antimicrobials, *Am. Rev. Respir. Dis. 84:*746–749 (1961).

158. Hagmar, B., Kutti, J., Lundin, P., Norlin, M., Weinfeld, A., and Wahlen, P., Disseminated infection caused by *Mycobacterium kansasii.* Report of a case and brief review of the literature, *Acta Med. Scand. 186:*93–99 (1969).

159. Hand, W. L., and Sanford, J. P., *Mycobacterium fortuitum*—A human pathogen, *Ann. Intern. Med. 73:*971–977 (1970).

160. Harrington, R., Jr., and Karlson, A. G., Destruction of various kinds of mycobacteria in milk by pasteurization, *Appl. Microbiol. 13:*494–495 (1965).

161. Hartwig, E. C., Cacciatore, E., and Dunbar, F. P., *M. fortuitum:* Its identification, incidence, and significance in Florida, *Am. Rev. Respir. Dis. 85:*84–91 (1962).

162. Hauduroy, P., Bel, F., and Hovanessian, A., Techniques permettant de faire un diagnostic précis de *Mycobactérium kansasii* (Hauduroy). *Ann. Inst. Pasteur* (Paris) *111:*84–86 (1966).

163. Hawkins, J. E., and McClean, V. R., Comparative studies of cycloserine inhibition of mycobacteria, *Am. Rev. Respir. Dis. 93:*594–602 (1966).

164. Hedgecock, L. W., and Blumenthal, H. T., The effect of isoniazid and para-aminosalicylic acid on infection in mice produced by *Mycobacterium kansasii, Am. Rev. Respir. Dis. 91:*21–29 (1965).

165. Hedstrom, H., Studies on so-called skin-tuberculosis in cattle: Concerning its prevalence in Sweden, its diagnosis, etiology, and allergy to tuberculin (monograph), Stockholm, 1949.

166. Hellerstrom, S., Ericsson, H., and Lagercrantz, R., Different types of swimming pool granuloma caused by mycobacteria, *Acta. Derm.–Venereol. 32:*249–256 (1956).

167. Hobby, G. L., Redmond, W. B., Runyon, E. H., Schaefer, W. B., Wayne, L. G., and Wichelshausen, R. H., A study on pulmonary disease associated with mycobacteria other than *Mycobacterium tuberculosis:* Identification and characterization of the mycobacteria. XVIII. A report of the Veterans Administration–Armed Forces Cooperative Study. *Am. Rev. Respir. Dis. 95:*954–971 (1967).

168. Honza, M., Kubin, M., Sikorova, A., and Janku, A., The effect of streptomycin and steroid hormones on evolution of experimental osteoarthritis caused by nonchromogenic mycobacteria, *Rozhledy v. Tuberk. av Nemocech Plicnich* (authors' abst. in Eng.) *24:*240–245 (1966).

169. Hsu, K. H. K., Nontuberculous mycobacterial infections in children, *J. Pediatr. 60:*705–710 (1962).

170. Humphriss, E., Peden, D., and Wright, H. D., The adequacy of commercial pasteurization for destruction of tubercle bacilli, *Lancet 1937-2:*151–152.

171. Inman, P. M., Beck, A., Brown, A. E., and Stanford, J. L., Outbreak of injection abscesses due to *Mycobacterium abscessus, Arch. Dermatol. 100:*141–147 (1969).

172. Jarnagin, J. L., Richards, W. D., Muhm, R. L., and Ellis, E. M., The isolation of *Mycobacterium xenopi* from granulomatous lesions of swine, *Am. Rev. Respir. Dis. 104:*763–765 (1971).

173. Jenkins, D. E., *in* Discussion, *Transactions of the 20th Research Conference on Pulmonary Disease,* p. 238 (1961).

174. Jenkins, D. E., Bahar, D., and Chofnas, I., Pulmonary disease due to atypical

mycobacteria: Current concepts, *Transactions of the 19th Conference on Chemotherapy of Tuberculosis*, pp. 224–229 (1960).

175. Jenkins, P. A., Marks, J., and Schaefer, W. B., Lipid chromatography and seroagglutination in the classification of rapidly growing mycobacteria, *Am. Rev. Respir. Dis. 103:*179–187 (1971).

176. Jenkins, P. A., Marks, J., and Schaefer, W. B., Thin-layer chromatography of mycobacterial lipids as an aid to classification. The scotochromogenic mycobacteria including *Mycobacterium scrofulaceum, Mycobacterium xenopi, Mycobacterium gordonae,* and *Mycobacterium flavescens, Tubercle 53:*118–127 (1972).

177. Jensen, K. A., and Lind, P., Specificity of purified tuberculins tested in guinea-pigs, *Acta. Tuberc. Scand. 17:*37–47 (1943).

178. Johanson, W. G., Jr., and Nicholson, D. P., Pulmonary disease due to *Mycobacterium kansasii:* An analysis of some factors affecting prognosis, *Am. Rev. Respir. Dis. 99:*73–85 (1969).

179. Jones, P. G., and Campbell, P. E., Tuberculous lymphadenitis in childhood: The significance of the anonymous mycobacteria, *Br. J. Surg. 50:*302–314 (1962).

180. Joos, H. A., Hilty, L. B., Courington, D., Schaefer, W. B., and Block, M., Fatal disseminated scotochromogenic mycobacteriosis in a child, *Am. Rev. Respir. Dis. 96:*795–801 (1967).

181. Judson, F. N., and Feldman, R. A., Mycobacterial skin tests in humans 12 years after infection with *Mycobacterium marinum, Am. Rev. Respir. Dis. 109:*544–547 (1974).

182. Justice, F. K., and Schwartz, W. S., Clinical characteristics of pulmonary infection associated with Battey-Bacilli. *Transactions of the 25th Research Conference on Pulmonary Disease*, pp. 83–86 (1966).

183. Kamat, S. R., Rossiter, C. E., and Gilson, J. C., A retrospective clinical study of pulmonary disease due to "anonymous mycobacteria" in Wales, *Thorax 16:*297–308 (1961).

184. Kane, R., and Vandivere, H. M., The significance of multiple simultaneous skin-testing in the prediction of various mycobacterial infections in the host, *Am. Rev. Respir. Dis. 105:*296–298 (1972).

185. Karassova, V., Weissfeiler, J., and Krasznay, E., Occurrence of atypical mycobacteria in *Macacus rhesus, Acta Microbiol. Acad. Sci. Hung. 12:*275–282 (1965).

186. Kasik, J. E., Monick, M., and Obstfeld, B., B-lactams, B-lactamase and Group III mycobacteria (abstr.), *Am. Rev. Respir. Dis. 115, No. 4, Part 2:*57 (1976).

187. Kazda, J., Mykobakterien in Trinkwasser als Ursache der Parallergie gegenüber Tuberkulinen bei Tieren, *Zentralbl. Bakteriol. Parasitenkd. Infektionskr. Hyg. Abt. 1 Orig. 203:*199–211 (1967).

188. Kazda, J., Die Bedeutung von Wasser für die Verbreitung von potentiell pathogenen Mykobakterien. 1. Möglichkeit für eine Vermehrung von Mykobakterien. *Zentralbl. Bakteriol. Parasitenkd. Infektionskr. Hyg. Erste Abt. Orig. Reihe B Hyg. Praev. Med. 158:*161–169 (1973).

189. Keller, R. H., and Runyon, E. H., Mycobacterial diseases, *Am. J. Roentgenol. Radium Ther. Nucl. Med. 92:*528–539 (1964).

190. Kelly, P. J., Weed, L. A., and Lipscomb, P. R., Infection of tendon sheaths, bursae, joints and soft tissues by acid-fast bacilli other than tubercle bacilli, *J. Bone J. Surg. Am. Vol. 45A:*327–336 (1963).

191. Kent, G., and Lester, W., Histopathology of human pulmonary disease produced by

photochromogenic mycobacteria, *Transactions of the 18th Conference on Chemotherapy of Tuberculosis*, pp. 241–245 (1959).

192. Kestle, D. G., Abbott, V. D., and Kubica, G. P., Differential identification of mycobacteria. II. Subgroups of Groups II and III (Runyon) with different clinical significance, *Am. Rev. Respir. Dis. 95:*1041–1042 (1967).

193. Kiewiet, A. A., and Thompson, J. E., Isolation of "atypical" mycobacteria from healthy individuals in tropical Australia, *Tubercle. 51:*296–299 (1970).

194. Kilbridge, T. M., Gonella, J. S., and Bolan, J. T., Pancytopenia and death. Disseminated anonymous mycobacterial infection, *Arch. Intern. Med. 120:*38–46 (1967).

195. Klinenberg, J. R., Grimley, P. M., and Seegmiller, J. E., Destructive polyarthritis due to a photochromogenic mycobacterium, *N. Engl. J. Med. 272:*190–193 (1965).

196. Kniker, W. T., The use of ion-exchange chromatography for mycobacterial antigen isolation, *Am. Rev. Respir. Dis. 92, Part 2 (Suppl.):*19–28 (1965).

197. Knox, J. M., Gever, S. G., Freeman, R. G., and Whitcomb, F., Atypical acid-fast infection of the skin, *Arch Dermatol. 84:*386–391 (1961).

198. Koenig, M. G., Collins, R. D., and Heyssel, R. M., Disseminated mycobacteriosis caused by Battey type mycobacteria, *Ann. Intern. Med. 64:*145–154 (1966).

199. Konno, K., Reliability of the niacin test, *Am. Rev. Respir. Dis. 82:*422–424 (1960).

200. Konyha, L. D., and Kreier, J. P., The significance of tuberculin tests in the horse, *Am. Rev. Respir. Dis. 103:*91–99 (1971).

201. Korn, O., Zur Kenntnis der säure-festen Bakterien, *Zentralbl. Bakteriol. Parasitenkd. Infektionskr. Hyg. Abt. 1 Orig. 25:*532–541 (1899).

202. Krasnow, I., and Gross, W., *Mycobacterium simiae* infection in the United States. A case report and discussion of the organism, *Am. Rev. Respir. Dis. 111:*357–360 (1975).

203. Krieg, R. E., Hochmeyer, W. T., and Connor, D. H., Toxin of *Mycobacterium ulcerans*. Production and effects in guinea pig skin, *Arch. Dermatol. 110:*783–788 (1974).

204. Krieger, I., Hahne, O. H., and Whitten, C. F., Atypical mycobacteria as a probable cause of chronic bone disease. A report of two cases, *J. Pediatr. 65:*340–349 (1964).

205. Kubica, G. P., Differential identification of atypical mycobacteria, *Am. Rev. Respir. Dis. 107:*9–21 (1973).

206. Kubica, G. P., Beam, R. E., Palmer, J. W., and Rigdon, R. L., The isolation of unclassified (atypical) acid-fast mycobacteria from soil and water samples collected in the State of Georgia, *Am. Rev. Respir. Dis. 88:*718–720 (1963).

207. Kubica, G. P., Gross, W. M., Hawkins, J. E., Sommers, H. M., Vestal, A. L., and Wayne, L. G., Laboratory services for mycobacterial diseases. *Am. Rev. Respir. Dis. 112:*773–787 (1975).

208. Kubica, G. P., and Vestal, A. L., The arylsulfatase activity of acid fast bacilli, *Am. Rev. Respir. Dis. 83:*728–732 (1961).

209. Kubin, M., Dvorsky, K., Eisnerova, R., Mesensky, I., Franc, K., and Matejka, M., Pulmonary and nonpulmonary disease in humans due to avian mycobacteria, *Am. Rev. Respir. Dis. 94:*31–39 (1966).

210. Kubin, M., Kruml., J., Horak, Z., Lukavsku, J., and Vanek, C., Pulmonary and nonpulmonary disease in humans due to avian mycobacteria. I. Clinical and epidemiological analysis of nine cases observed in Czechoslovakia, *Am. Rev. Respir. Dis. 94:*20–30 (1966).

211. Kubin, M., Matsukova, E., and Kazda, J., *Mycobacterium brunense*, n. sp., identified

as sero-type Davis of Group III mycobacteria, *Zentralbl. Bakteriol. Parasitenkd. Infectionskr. Hyg. Abt. 1 Orig. 210:*207–211 (1969).

212. Kuo, T., and Roshi, J., Granulomatous inflammation in spleenectomy specimens. Clinico-pathologic study of 20 cases, *Arch. Pathol. 98:*261–268 (1974).

213. Kushner, D. S., McMillen, S., and Senderi, M., Atypical acid-fast bacilli: II. *Mycobacterium fortuitum:* Bacteriological characteristics and pathogenicity for laboratory animals, *Am. Rev. Tuberc. Pulm. Dis. 76:*108–122 (1957).

214. Lakshminarayan, S., and Sahn, S., Disseminated infection caused by *Mycobacterium avium*—Report of a case associated with leucopenia, *Am. Rev. Respir. Dis. 108:*123–126 (1973).

215. Larson, C. L., Baker, M. B., Baker, R., and Ribi, E., Study of delayed reactions using protoplasm from acid-fast bacilli as provoking antigen, *Am. Rev. Respir. Dis. 94:*257–259 (1966).

216. Larson, C. L., and Wicht., W. C., Resistance to infection with virulent tubercle bacilli in mice immunized with *Mycobacterium balnei* and unclassified mycobacteria administered aerogenically, *Am. Rev. Respir. Dis. 88:*456–461 (1963).

217. Lavalle Aguilar, P., Marquez Ituribarria, F., and Middlebrook, G., Un caso de infeccion humana por *Mycobacterium ulcerans* en el hemisferio occidentale nota praevia, *Int. J. Lepr. 21:*469–476 (1953).

218. Law, S. W., Surgical treatment of atypical mycobacterial disease, *Dis. Chest 47:*296–303 (1965).

219. Lefkowitz, L., Sanford, J. P., and Chapman, J. S., Skin tests with "Tuberculins" prepared from atypical mycobacteria (abst.), *Clin. Res. 8:*56 (1966).

220. Lesslie, J. W., and Zorawski, C. M., Yield and specificity of tuberculin PPD derived from four strains of *Mycobacterium avium* and a comparison of some antigenic properties of these strains, *Tubercle 50:*42–50 (1969).

221. Lester, W., Unclassified mycobacterial disease, *Am. Rev. Med. 17:*351–360 (1966).

222. Lester, W., Botkin, K., and Colton, R., Analysis of 49 cases of pulmonary disease caused by photochromogenic mycobacteria, *Transactions of the 19th Conference on Chemotherapy of Tuberculosis*, pp. 289–297 (1958).

223. Levine, R. A., Infection of the orbit by an atypical mycobacterium, *Arch. Ophthalmol. 82:*608–610 (1969).

224. Lewis, A. G., Lasche, E. M., Armstrong, A. L., and Dunbar, F. P., A clinical study of the chronic lung disease due to nonphotochromogenic acid-fast bacilli, *Ann. Intern. Med. 53:*273–285 (1960).

225. Lincoln, E. M., and Gilbert, L. A., Disease in children due to mycobacteria other than *Mycobacterium tuberculosis, Am. Rev. Respir. Dis. 105:*683–714 (1972).

226. Lind, A., Serological studies of mycobacteria by means of diffusion-in-gel techniques, Dissertation, Goteberg, 1961.

227. Lind, A., and Norlin, M., A comparative serological study *M. avium, M. ulcerans, M. balnei*, and *M. marinum* by means of double diffusion-in-gel methods. A preliminary investigation, *Scand. J. Clin. Lab. Invest. 15, Suppl. 69:*152–163 (1963).

228. Lindo, S. D., and Daniels, F., Jr., Buruli ulcer in New York City, *J. Amer. Med. Assoc. 228:*1138–1139 (1974).

229. Linell, F., and Norden, A., *Mycobacterium balnei*—A new acid-fast bacillus occurring in swimming pools and capable of producing skin lesions in humans, *Acta Tuberc. Scand. Suppl. 33:*1–84 (1954).

230. Listwan, W. J., Roth, D. A., Tsung, S. H., and Rose, H. D., Disseminated *Mycobac-*

terium kansasii infection with pancytopenia and interstitial nephritis, *Ann. Intern. Med.* *83:*70–73 (1975).

231. Lorian, V., Direct cord reading medium for isolation of mycobacteria, *Appl. Microbiol. 14:*603–607 (1966).

232. Lorian, V., and Finland, M., *In vitro* effect of rifampin on mycobacteria, *Appl. Microbiol. 17:*202–207 (1969).

233. MacCallum, P., Tolhurst, J. C., Buckle, C., and Sissons, H. A., A new mycobacterial infection in man, *J. Pathol. Bacteriol. 60:*93–122 (1948).

234. Magnusson, M., Specificity of sensitins. III. Further studies in guinea pigs with sensitins of various species of *Mycobacterium* and *Nocardia, Am. Rev. Respir. Dis. 86:*395–404 (1962).

235. Magnusson, M., Bleiker, M. A., and Griep, W. A., Comparative intradermal reactions of young Dutch males to purified tuberculin (PPD) and other sensitins. I. Observations with different mycobacterial sensitins in non-vaccinated persons, *Acta Tuberc. Scand. 42:*53–72 (1962).

236. Mallman, W. L., Mallman, V. H., and Ray, J. A., Mycobacteriosis in swine caused by atypical mycobacteria, *Proceedings of the U.S. Livestock Sanitary Association,* pp. 180–183 (1962).

237. Mallman, W. L., Mallman, V. H., Ray, J. A., McGavin, M. D., and Ellis, D. L., Infectivity of atypical Group III mycobacteria of NGL cattle, swine, and soil origin, *Scientific Proceedings of the 100th Annual Meeting of the American Veterinary Medicine Association,* pp. 265–267 (1963).

238. Mankiewicz, E., Agar diffusion precipitation and complement fixation tests applied to the study of the antigenic relationships between chromogenic acid-fast mycobacteria and *Mycobacterium tuberculosis, Can. J. Microbiol. 4:*565–570 (1958).

239. Mankiewicz, E., Mycobacteriophages isolated from persons with tuberculous and non-tuberculous conditions, *Nature (London) 191:*1416–1417 (1961).

240. Marks, J., "Opportunist" mycobacteria in England and Wales, *Tubercle Suppl. 50:*78–80 (1969).

241. Marks, J., and Birn, K. J., Infection due to *Mycobacterium avium, Br. Med. J. 1963-2:*1503–1506.

242. Marks, J., Jenkins, P. A., and Tsukamura, M., *Mycobacterium szulgai*—A new pathogen, *Tubercle 53:*210–214 (1972).

243. Marks, J., and Richards, M., Classification of the anonymous mycobacteria as a guide to their significance, *Mon. Bull. Minist. Health Public Health Lab. Serv. Directed Med. Res. Counc. 21:*200–208 (1963).

244. Marks, J., and Schwabacher, H., Infection due to *Mycobacterium xenopei, Br. Med. J. 1:*32–33 (1965).

245. Marks, J., and Szulga, T., Thin-layer chromatography of mycobacterial lipids as an aid to classification: Technical procedures: *Mycobacterium fortuitum, Tubercle 46:*400–411 (1965).

246. McCracken, G. H., Jr., and Reynolds, R. C., Primary lymphopenic immunologic deficiency. Disseminated *Mycobacterium kansasii* infection, *Am. J. Dis. Child. 120:*143–147 (1970).

247. McCusker, J. J., and Green, R. A., Generalized nontuberculous mycobacteriosis, *Am. Rev. Respir. Dis. 86:*405–414 (1962).

248. Medd, W. E., and Hayhoe, F. G. J., Tuberculous miliary necrosis with pancytopenia, *Q. J. Med. 24:*351–364 (1955).

249. Meissner, G., and Schröder, K.-H., Relationship between *Mycobacterium simiae* and *Mycobacterium habana, Am. Rev. Respir. Dis. 111:*196–200 (1975).

250. Merckx, J. J., Karlson, A. G., and Carr, D. T., Disease in man associated with unclassified acid-fast mycobacteria, *Proc. Staff Meetings Mayo Clin. 38:*271–279 (1963).

251. Merckx, J. J., Soule, E. H., and Karlson, A. G., The histopathology of lesions caused by unclassified acid-fast bacteria in man, *Am. J. Clin. Pathol. 41:*244–255 (1964).

252. Meyer, K. F., Specific paratuberculous enteritis of cattle in America, *J. Med. Res. 29:*147–165 (1913).

253. Middlebrook, G., Isoniazid resistance and catalase activity of tubercle bacilli, *Am. Rev. Tuberc. Pulm. Dis. 69:*471–472 (1954).

254. Middlebrook, G., Cohn, M. L., and Oestreicher, R., Chromogenic acid-fast bacilli from human sources, *Am. Rev. Tuberc. Pulm. Dis. 72:*693 (1955).

255. Moeller, A., Mikroörganismen, die den Tuberkelbacillen verwandt sind und bei Thieren eine miliäre Tuberkelkrankheit verursachen, *Dtsch. Med. Wochenschr. 1898, No. 24:*376–379.

256. Moeller, A., Ein neuer säure- und alcohol-fester Bacillus aus der Tuberkelbacillengruppe welche echte Verzweigungsformen bildet, *Zentralbl. Bakteriol. Parasitenkd. Infektionskr. Hyg. Abt. 1 Orig. 25:*369–373 (1899).

257. Moeller, A., Zur Verbreitungsweise der Tuberkelpilze, *Z. Hyg. Infektionskr. 32:*205–213 (1899).

258. Moeller, A., Die Beziehungen des Tuberkelbacillus zu den anderen säurefesten Bakterien und zu den Strahlenpilzen, *Zentralbl. Bakteriol. Parasitenkd. Infektionskr. Hyg. Abt. 1 Orig. 30:*513–523 (1901).

259. Moeller, A., Die Behandlung der Tuberkulos mit kaltbluter Bakterien (Blindschleichen-Vakzine) *Tuberkulosearzt 13:*205–210 (1914).

260. Mohler, J. H., and Washburn, H. J., The susceptibility of tubercle bacilli to modification, *Bureau of Animal Industry 23rd Annual Report 1906:*113–163.

261. Molavi, A., and Weinstein, L., In-vitro activity of erythromycin against atypical mycobacteria, *J. Infect. Dis. 123:*216–219 (1971).

262. Möllers, B., Zur Frage der Tuberkeloseinfektion des Menschen durch Perlsuchtbazillen, *Dtsch. Med. Wochenschr 36:*204–207 (1910).

263. Mollohan, C. S., and Romer, M. S., Public health significance of swimming pool granuloma, *Am. J. Public Health 51:*883–891 (1961).

264. Morris, C. A., Grant, G. H., Everall, P. H., and Myres, A. T. M., Tuberculoid lymphadenitis due to *Mycobacterium chelonei, J. Clin. Pathol. (London) 26:*422–426 (1973).

265. Newman, H., Renal disease associated with atypical mycobacteria: Battey type. Case Report, *J. Urol. 103:*403–405 (1970).

266. Nicholson, D. P., and Sevier, W. R., *Mycobacterium fortuitum* as a pathogen. A case report, *Am. Rev. Respir. Dis. 104:*747–750 (1971).

267. Nissen-Meyer, S., Epidemiologic studies of tuberculin sensitivity. III. Estimation of prevalence of mycobacterial infection from results of skin tests with mycobacterial antigens, *Am. J. Hyg. 72:*169–194 (1960).

268. Noufflard, H., and Berteaux, S., Activité anti-tuberculeuse de produit B-663, *Ann. Inst. Pasteur* (Paris) *95:*449–455 (1958).

269. Olsovsky, V., Mikova, V., Kubin, M., (Title of paper in Czech; authors' abstract in English.) *Cesk. Epidemiol. Mikrobiol. Imunol. 21:*20–25 (1972).

270. O'Reilly, L. M., and MacClancey, B. N., Tuberculosis—Dual infections in a dairy herd due to avian and bovine type bacilli, *Ir. Vet. J. 22:*222–230 (1968). (Abst. from *Veterinary Bull.* No. 325).

271. Organick, A. B., Ingersol, R. L., and Bitner, L. M., Disseminated disease due to a photochromogenic mycobacterium with comments on chemotherapy with INH, SM, PAS, and erythromycin, *Transactions of the 19th Conference on Chemotherapy of Tuberculosis,* pp. 234–235 (1960).

272. Ouchterlony, O., Antigen–antibody reactions in gels. IV. Types of reactions in coordinated systems of diffusion, *Acta Pathol. Microbiol. Scand. 32:*231–240 (1953).

273. Owen, D. S., Jr., and Toone, E., Soft tissue infection by Group I atypical mycobacteria, *South Med. J. 63:*116–117 (1970).

274. Owen, M., Smith, A., and Coultras, J., Granulomatous lesions occurring at site of injections of vaccines and antibiotics, *South Med. J. 56:*949–962 (1963).

275. Owens, D. W., and McBride, M. E., Sporotrichoid cutaneous infection with *Mycobacterium kansasii, Arch. Dermatol. 100:*54–58 (1969).

276. Palmer, C. E., Edwards, L. B., Hopwood, L., and Edwards, P. Q., Experimental and epidemiological basis for the interpretation of skin test sensitivity, *J. Pediatr. 55:*413–429 (1959).

277. Palmer, C. E., and Hopwood, L., Effect of previous infection with unclassified mycobacteria on survival of guinea-pigs challenged with virulent tubercle bacilli, *Bull. Int. Union Tuberc. 32:*398–402 (1962).

278. Palmer, C. E., and Long, M. W., Effects of infection with atypical mycobacteria on BCG vaccination and tuberculins, *Am. Rev. Respir. Dis. 94:*553–568 (1966).

279. Pappenheim, A., Befund von Smegmabacillen im menschlichen Lungenaufwurf, *Berl. Klin. Wochenschr. 35:*809–813 (1898).

280. Parlett, R., and Youmans, G. P., Antigenic relationships between mycobacteria as determined by agar diffusion precipitin technique, *Am. Rev. Tuberc. Pulm. Dis. 73:*637–649 (1956).

281. Parlett, R., and Youmans, G. P., Antigenic relationships between ninety-eight strains of mycobacteria using agar gel-diffusion precipitation techniques, *Am. Rev. Tuberc. Pulm. Dis. 77:*450–461 (1958).

282. Parlett, R., Youmans, G. P., Rehr, C., and Lester, W., The detection of antibodies in the serum of tuberculous patients by an agar double-diffusion precipitation technique, *Am. Rev. Tuberc. Pulm. Dis. 77:*462–472 (1958).

283. Patterson, A. B., Stuart, P., Lesslie, I. W., and Leech, F. B., The use of tests on slaughterhouse cattle for estimating potencies of tuberculins and for the calculation of discrimination tests, *J. Hyg. 56:*1–18 (1958).

284. Pergament, M., Gonzales, R., and Fraley, E. E., Atypical mycobacteriosis of the urinary tract. A case of extensive disease caused by the Battey bacillus, *J. Amer. Med. Assoc. 229:*816–817 (1974).

285. Petroff, S. A., and Steenken, W., Jr., Biological studies of saprophytic acid fast organisms: 1. Dissociation of *Mycobacterium phlei, J. Infect. Dis. 56:*277–287 (1935).

286. Pfuetze, K. H., Van Vo, L., Reimann, A. F., Berg, G. S., and Lester, W., Photochromogenic mycobacterial pulmonary disease, *Am. Rev. Respir. Dis. 92:*470–475 (1965).

287. Phillips, S., and Larkin, J. C., Jr., Atypical pulmonary tuberculosis caused by unclassified mycobacteria, *Ann. Intern. Med. 60:*401–408 (1964).

288. Philpott, J. A., Jr., Woodburn, A. R., Philpott, O. S., Schaefer, W. B., and Mollohan, C. S., Swimming pool granuloma, *Arch. Dermatol. 88:*158–162 (1963).
289. Pinner, M., Atypical acid-fast organisms, *Proc. Soc. Exp. Biol. Med. 30:*214–216 (1932).
290. Pinner, M., Atypical acid-fast organisms: III. Chromogenic acid-fast bacilli from human lungs, *Am. Rev. Tuberc. Pulm. Dis. 32:*424–439 (1935).
291. Pinner, M., Atypical acid-fast organisms. IV. Smooth-growing tubercle bacilli, *Am. Rev. Tuberc. Pulm. Dis. 32:*440–445 (1935).
292. Pope, J. W., Ponce, L., and Medina, M., Surgical treatment in pulmonary infections due to atypical mycobacterium (sic), *Am. J. Surg. 114:*739–743 (1967).
293. Porres, J. M., Isolation of *Mycobacterium rhodochrous* from a cutaneous lesion, *Arch. Dermatol. 108:*411–412 (1973).
294. Potts, W. E., and Chapman, J. S., Reversion of tuberculin test in no-contact children (Abst.) *Am. Rev. Respir. Dis. 86:*123 (1962).
295. Prather, E. C., Bond, J. O., Hartwig, E. C., and Dunbar, F. P., Preliminary report: Epidemiology of infections due to atypical acid-fast bacilli, *Dis. Chest 39:*129–139 (1961).
296. Prissick, F. H., and Masson, A. M., Cervical lymphadenitis in children caused by chromogenic mycobacteria, *Can. Med. Assoc. J. 75:*798–802 (1956).
297. Pust, R. E., Onubugu, H. O. N., Egornu, L. I., and Smithwick, R., Pulmonary disease due to *Mycobacterium fortuitum* in a Nigerian, *Am. Rev. Respir. Dis. 108:*1416–1420 (1973).
298. Rabinowitsch, L., Zur Frage des Vorkommens von Tuberkel-bacillen in Markt-butter, *Z. Hyg. Infektionskr. 26:*90–111 (1897).
299. Rabinowitsch, L., Der Infectiosität der Milch tuberkuloser Kuhe, die Sicherstollung der Bakteriologischen Diagnose, sowie die praktische Bedeutung des Tuberculins für Ausrottlung der Rindertuberculose, *Z. Hyg. Infektionskr. 37:*439–448 (1901).
300. Race, G. J., in "The Anonymous Mycobacteria in Human Disease" (J. S. Chapman, Ed.), pp. 37–44, Charles C Thomas, Springfield, Ill. (1960).
301. Reback, J. F., Atypical mycobacteria, particularly in relation to lesions of the extremities, *M. Soc. Med. Technol. News Letter* February, 1963 (no pagination).
302. Reid, I. S., *Mycobacterium ulcerans* infection: A report of 13 cases at the Port Moresby General Hospital, *Med. J. Aust. 1967–1:*427–431.
303. Reid, J. D., and Wolinsky, E., Histopathology of lymphadenitis caused by atypical mycobacteria, *Am. Rev. Respir. Dis. 99:*8–12 (1969).
304. Reimann, H. A., and Chun Ma, P. P., Dissociants of *M. tuberculosis* and atypical mycobacteria, *Am. Rev. Respir. Dis. 92:*193–209 (1965).
305. Reiner, E., Hicks, J. J., Beam, R. E., and David, H. L., Recent studies in mycobacterial differentiation by means of pyrolysis gas–liquid chromatography, *Am. Rev. Respir. Dis. 104:*656–660 (1971).
306. Rheins, M. S., Burrell, R. G., and Birkeland, J. M., Tuberculous antibodies demonstrated by agar diffusion, *Am. Rev. Tuberc. Pulm. Dis. 74:*229–238 (1956).
307. Revill, W. D. L., and Barker, D. J. P., Seasonal distribution of mycobacterial skin ulcers, *Br. J. Prev. Soc. Med. 26:*23–27 (1972).
308. Reznikov, M., Leggo, J. H., and Dawson, D. J., Investigation by sero-agglutination of strains of *Mycobacterium intracellulare–Mycobacterium scrofulaceum* group from house dusts and sputum in southeastern Queensland, *Am. Rev. Respir. Dis. 104:*951–953 (1971).

309. Richmond, L., and Cummings, M. M., An evaluation of the methods of testing for virulence of acid-fast bacilli, *Am. Rev. Tuberc. Pulm. Dis. 62:*632–637 (1950).

310. Robakiewicz, M., and Grzybowski, S., Epidemiological aspects of non-tuberculous mycobacterial disease and of tuberculosis in British Columbia, *Am. Rev. Respir. Dis. 109:*613–620 (1974).

311. Rosenzweig, D. Y., Course and long-term follow-up of 100 cases of pulmonary infection due to *M. avium* (Abst.) *Am. Rev. Respir. Dis. 113, No. 4, Part 2:*55 (1976).

312. Runyon, E. H., Anonymous mycobacteria in pulmonary disease, *Med. Clin. North Am. 43:*273–290 (1959).

313. Runyon, E. H., *Mycobacterium intracellulare, Am. Rev. Respir. Dis. 95:*861–865 (1967).

314. Runyon, E. H., When mycobacteria and mycobacteriosis? (Editorial), *Ann. Intern. Med. 75:*467–468 (1971).

315. Runyon, E. H., and Dietz, T. M., Skin sensitivity in guinea pigs produced by Group II mycobacteria, *Am. Rev. Respir. Dis. 104:*107–113 (1971).

316. Rynearson, T. K., Shronts, J. S., and Wolinsky, E., Rifampin: *In vitro* effect on atypical mycobacteria, *Am. Rev. Respir. Dis. 104:*272–274 (1971).

317. Saito, H., Hosokawa, H., and Tasaka, H., The heat stable phosphatase activity of mycobacteria, *Am. Rev. Respir. Dis. 97:*474–476 (1968).

318. Saito, H., and Kubica, G. P., Serological studies of avian–Group III nonphotochromogen complex by agglutination, *Am. Rev. Respir. Dis. 98:*47–59 (1968).

319. Saito, H., *et al.* (sic), A case of preauricular and cervical lymphadenitis due to *M. intracellulare, Kekkaku 47:*29–35 (1972). Abst. in *Am. Rev. Respir. Dis. 106:*352 (1972).

320. Saito, H., Tasaka, H., Osasa, S., Yamura, T., Fukuhara, T., and Yamada, A., Disseminated *Mycobacterium intracellulare* infection, *Am. Rev. Respir. Dis. 109:*572–576 (1974).

321. Salyer, K. E., Votteler, T. P., and Dorman, G. W., Surgical management of cervical adenitis due to atypical mycobacteria in children, *J. Amer. Med. Assoc. 204:*1037–1040 (1968).

322. Scammon, L. A., Pickett, M. J., Froman, S., and Will, D. W., Non-chromogenic acid-fast bacilli isolated from tuberculous swine: Their relation to *M. avium* and the "Battey" type of unclassified mycobacteria, *Am. Rev. Respir. Dis. 87:*97–102 (1963).

323. Schachter, E. M., Tuberculin-negative tuberculosis, *Am. Rev. Respir. Dis. 106:*587–593 (1972).

324. Schaefer, W. B., Serologic identification and classification of atypical mycobacteria by their agglutination, *Am. Rev. Respir. Dis. 92, Part 2 (Suppl.):*85–93 (1965).

325. Schaefer, W. B., Incidence of serotypes of *Mycobacterium avium* and atypical mycobacteria in human and animal diseases, *Am. Rev. Respir. Dis. 97:*18–23 (1968).

326. Schaefer, W. B., Birn, K. J., Jenkins, P. A., and Marks, J., Infection with the avian-Battey group of mycobacteria in England and Wales, *Br. Med. J. 1969-2:*412–415.

327. Schaefer, W. B., Wolinsky, E., Jenkins, P. A., and Marks, J., *Mycobacterium szulgai*—A new pathogen: Serological identification and report of five new cases, *Am. Rev. Respir. Dis. 108:*1320–1326 (1973).

328. Schepers, G. W., Smart, R. H., Smith, C. R., Dworski, M., and Delahant, A. B., Fatal silicosis with complicating infection by an atypical acid-fast photochromogenic bacillus, *Ind. Med. Surg. 27:*27–36 (1958).

329. Schmidt, J. D., Yeager, H., Jr., Smith, E. B., and Raleigh, J. W., Cutaneous infection due to a Runyon Group III atypical mycobacterium, *Am. Rev. Respir. Dis. 106:*469–471 (1972).

330. Schonell, M. E., Crofton, J. W., Stuart, A. E., and Wallace A., Disseminated infection with *Mycobacterium avium:* Part 1—Clinical features, treatment and pathology, *Tubercle 49:*12–30 (1968).

331. Schröder, K.-H., Investigation into the relationship of *M. ulcerans* to *M. buruli* and other mycobacteria, *Am. Rev. Respir. Dis. 111:*559–562 (1975).

332. Schwabacher, A., A strain of mycobacterium isolated from skin lesions of a cold-blooded animal, *Xenopus laevis,* and its relation to atypical acid-fast bacilli occurring in man, *J. Hyg. 57:*57–67 (1957).

333. Selkon, J. B., "Atypical Mycobacteria"—A review, *Tubercle 50 (Suppl.):*70–77 (1969).

334. Selkon, J. B., and Mitchison, D. A., Atypical mycobacteria and drug-resistant tubercle bacilli isolated during a survey of untreated patients with pulmonary tuberculosis, *Tubercle 40:*141–154 (1959).

335. Shimoide, H., Clinical study of atypical mycobacterial infection. III. Disease caused by *Mycobacterium kansasii, Jap. J. Tuberc. Chest Dis. 30:*128–134 (1971). Abst. in *Am. Rev. Respir. Dis. 104:*152 (1971).

336. Shimoide, H., Clinical study of mycobacterioses. V. Disease caused by *M. kansasii* in Japan, *Jap. J. Tuberc. Chest Dis. 31:*924–936 (1972). Abst. in *Am. Rev. Respir. Dis. 107:*709 (1973).

337. Singer, E., Nonspecific sensitization to old tuberculin: Asymptomatic infection with mycobacteria, *Tubercle 46:*270–272 (1965).

338. Smith, D. T., and Johnston, W. W., Single and multiple infections with atypical mycobacteria, *Am. Rev. Respir. Dis. 90:*899–912 (1964).

339. Smith, D. T., Johnston, W. W., Cain, I. M., and Schumacher, M., Changes in tuberculin pattern in students between 1930 and 1960, *Am. Rev. Respir. Dis. 83:*213–234 (1961).

340. Smith, D. W., Grover, A. A., and Wiegeshaus, E., Nonliving immunogenic substances of mycobacteria, *Adv. Tuberc. Res. 16:*191–227 (1968).

341. Smith, D. W., and Randall, H. M., Mycosides of mycobacteria, *Am. Rev. Respir. Dis. 92, Suppl. 34:*34–41 (1965).

342. Smith, D. W., Randall, H. M., MacLennan, A. P., Putney, R. K., and Rao, S. V., Detection of specific lipids in mycobacteria by infrared spectroscopy, *J. Bacteriol. 79:*217–229 (1960).

343. Smith, T., The relation between human and animal tuberculosis with special reference to the question of transformation of human and other types of the tubercle bacillus, *Boston Med. Surg. J. 159:*707–711 (1908).

344. Smyth, J. T., Kovacs, N., and Harris, W. P., Pulmonary disease due to unclassified mycobacteria (Battey-type): Report of 14 cases with histological confirmation, *Tubercle 45:*223–228 (1964).

345. Snijder, J., Histopathology of primary lesions caused by atypical mycobacteria, *J. Pathol Bacteriol. 98:*65–73 (1965).

346. Spengler, C., Ein neues immunisierndes Heilverfahren der Lungenschwinsucht mit Perlsucht-tuberculin, *Dtsch. Med. Wochenschr. 1905, No. 31:*1228–1230.

347. Spengler, C., Neue Farbemethoden fur Perlsucht- und Tuberkel-bacillen und deren Differential-diagnose, *Dtsch. Med. Wochenschr. 33:*337–338 (1907).

348. Stadnichenko, A. S. M., Sweany, H. C., and Kloeck, J. M., Types of tubercle bacilli in birds and mammals: Their incidence, isolation and identification, *Am. Rev. Tuberc. Pulm. Dis.* *51:*276–293 (1945).

349. Stafseth, H. J., Buggar, R. J., Thompson, W. H., and Nev, L., The cultivation and egg-transmission of the avian tubercle bacillus, *J. Am. Vet. Med. Assoc.* *85:*342 (1934). Abst. in *Am. Rev. Tuberc. Pulm. Dis.* *32:*8 (1935).

350. Stanford, J. L., and Beck, A., An antigenic analysis of the mycobacteria, *Mycobacterium fortuitum, Mycobacterium kansasii, Mycobacterium phlei, Mycobacterium smegmatis,* and *Mycobacterium tuberculosis, J. Pathol. Bacteriol.* *95:*131–139 (1968).

351. Stanford, J. L., and Gunthorpe, W. J., Serological and bacteriological investigation of *Mycobacterium ranae (fortuitum), J. Bacteriol.* *98:*373–383 (1969).

352. Steenken, W., Jr., and Landau, A., Dissociation of two unusual acid-fast organisms isolated from human sources, *J. Infect. Dis.* *58:*247–258 (1936).

353. Steenken, W., Jr., and Smith, M. M., Culture of tubercle bacilli. 1. The effect of sodium hydroxide and sulfuric acid upon acid-fast variants of homologous strains and the influence of the hydrogen ion concentration of different media upon subsequent growth, *Am. Rev. Tuberc. Pulm. Dis.* *38:*503–513 (1938).

354. Steingrube, V. A., Murphy, D., McMahon, S., Chapman, J. S., and Nash, D. R., The effect of metal ions on the atypical mycobacteria. Growth and colony coloration, *Zentralbl. Bakteriol. Parasitenkd. Infektionskr. Hyg. Abt. 1 Orig.* *230:*223–236 (1975).

355. Stewart, C. J., Dixon, J. M. S., and Curtis, B. A., Isolation of mycobacteria from tonsils, nasopharyngeal secretions and lymph nodes, *Tubercle 51:*178–183 (1970).

356. Stottmeier, K. D., Tose, L., and Jones, C., Clinical and bacteriological evaluation of pulmonary mycobacteriosis in the Greater Boston area, *Am. Rev. Respir. Dis.* *108:*1227–1230 (1973).

357. Straus, I., and Dubarry, A., Récherches sur la durée de la vie des microbes pathogènes dans l'eau, *Arch. Med. Exp. Anat. Pathol. 1889–1:*5, from Rosenau, *Internatl. Cong. Against Tuberc. 1, Part 1:*43.

358. Sula, L., Stott, H., Kubin, M., and Kiaer, J., A study of mycobacteria isolated from cervical lymph nodes of African patients in Kenya, *Bull. W.H.O.* *23:*613–634 (1960).

359. Tacquet, A., Andrejew, A., and Tison, F., Notions récentes sur le pouvoir pathogène des mycobactéries atypiques pour l'animal, *Zentralbl. Bakteriol. Parasitenkd. Infektionskr. Hyg. Abt. 1 Orig.* I Referate, *194:*236–237 (1964).

360. Tacquet, A., Collet, A., Devulder, B., and Martin, J. C., Action of certain antibacillary substances in the experimental infection of guinea-pigs exposed to dust by *Mycobacterium kansasii, Z. Tuberkulose Erkr. Thoraxorgane 127:*127–131 (1967).

361. Tacquet, A., Collet, A., Macquet, V., Martin, J. C., Gernez-Rieux, C., and Policard, A., Étude expérimentale de l'influence d'empoussierage du poumon sur son infection par les mycobactéries atypiques, *C. R. Acad. Sci.* (Paris) *257:*3103–3105 (1963).

362. Tacquet, A., Devulder, B., and Tison, F., Frequency and evolutive aspects of pulmonary and ganglionary mycobacterioses in northern France, *Z. Tuberkulose Erkr. Thoraxorgane 127:*93–99 (1967).

363. Tacquet, A., Devulder, B., Tison, F., and Martin, J. C., Traitement de l'infection expérimentale a *Mycobactérium kansasii* du cobaye pneumoconiotique. Intérêt de la 4-4- di-isoamyl oxythiocarbanilide, *Ann. Inst. Pasteur* (Lille) *18:*95–107 (1967).

364. Tacquet, A., Guillaume, J., Tison, F., and Kuperwasser, B., Identification de l'espèce

Mycobacterium pellegrino par l'étude de certains derivés nitrés, *Ann. Inst. Pasteur* (Lille) *12:*221–223 (1960).

365. Tacquet, A., and Tison, F., Techniques courantes d'identification des mycobactéries atypiques, *Pathol. Biol. 9:*1185–1188 (1961).

366. Tacquet, A., Tison, F., and Devulder, B., Les variétés scotochromogènes de *Mycobacterium kansasii.* Étude bactériologique et biochimique, *Ann. Inst. Pasteur* (Paris) *108:*514–525 (1965).

367. Tacquet, A., Tison, F., and Devulder, B., Quelques aspects actuels des infections bronchopulmonaires provoquées par les mycobactéries dites "atypiques," *Rev. Tuberc. Pneumol. 28:*89–116 (1964).

368. Tacquet, A., Tison, F., Devulder, B., and Roos, P., Techniques de récherche des mycobactéries dans le lait et les produits laitiers. Incidences pratiques sur la prophlaxie de la tuberculose bovine at de l'epidemiologie des mycobactérioses humaines, *Ann. Inst. Pasteur* (Lille) *17:*161–171 (1966).

369. Tacquet, A., Tison, F., Devulder, B., and Roos, P., Les récherches des mycobactéries dans les boues de centrifugation industrielle du lait de vache, *Ann. Inst. Pasteur* (Lille) *17:*173–179 (1966).

370. Tacquet, A., Tison, F., Roos, P., and Devulder, B., Qualitative study of the lipase and B-D-galactosidase activities of mycobacteria, *Z. Tuberkulose Erkr. Thoraxorgane 127:*37–40 (1967).

371. Takeya, K., Zinnaka, Y., Yamaura, K., and Toda, T., Bacteriophage susceptibility and tuberculin specificity of unclassified mycobacteria, *Am. Rev. Respir. Dis. 81:*674–682 (1960).

372. Takeya, K., Nakayama, Y., and Nakayama, H., Relationship between *Mycobacterium fortuitum* and *Mycobacterium runyonii*, *Am. Rev. Respir. Dis. 96:*532–535 (1967).

373. Tammemagi, L., and Simmons, G. C., Battey-type mycobacterial infection of pigs, *Aust. Vet. J. 44:*121 (1963).

374. Tanzil, H. O. K., Chatim, A., Kurniawan, A. S., and Hasrul, H., The inhibitory action of nitroxiline on different mycobacteria and nocardia, *Am. Rev. Respir. Dis. 105:*455–456 (1972).

375. Tasaka, H., *et al.* (sic), Two cases of pulmonary disease caused by *Mycobacterium chelonei, Jap. J. Tuberc. Chest Dis. 31:*515–519 (1972). Abst. in *Am. Rev. Respir. Dis. 106:*815 (1972).

376. Thurston, J. R., and Steenken, W., Jr., Comparison of gel precipitin and sensitized erythrocyte techniques for the detection of antibody in the serum of tuberculous and nontuberculous patients, *Am. Rev. Respir. Dis. 81:*695–703 (1960).

377. Timpe, A., and Runyon, E. H., Relationship of "atypical" acid-fast bacilli to human disease: Preliminary report, *J. Lab. Clin. Med. 44:*202–209 (1954).

378. Tison, F., Devulder, B., Roos, P., and Tacquet, A., Techniques et resultats de la récherche des mycobactéries dan les viandes, *Ann. Inst. Pasteur* (Lille) *17:*156–160 (1966).

379. Tison, F., Tacquet, A., and Devulder, B., Récherche des mycobactéries dans les eaux des piscines et les eaux usées de la région du nord, *Ann. Inst. Pasteur* (Lille) *18:*167–176 (1967).

380. Tobie, W. C., "*Mycobacterium tuberculosis* No. 607" and similar doubtful tubercle bacilli, A review, *Am. Rev. Tuberc. Pulm. Dis. 58:*693–697 (1948).

381. Tobler, M., Beitrag zur Frage des Vorkommens von Tuberkelbacillen und anderen säurefesten Bacillen der Marktbutter, *Z. Hyg. Infektionskr. Hyg. 36:*120–150 (1901).

382. Tolhurst, J. C., Buckle, G., and Wellington, N. A. M., The experimental infection of calves with *Mycobacterium ulcerans*, *J. Hyg. 57:*47–56 (1959).

383. Tsai, S. H., Yue, W. Y., and Duthoy, E. J., Roentgen aspects of chronic pulmonary mycobacteriosis. An analysis of 18 cases, including one with renal involvement, *Radiology 90:*306–310 (1968).

384. Tsang, A. Y., Bentz, R. R., Schork, M. A., and Sodeman, T. M., Combined versus single drug susceptibility studies of *M. kansasii* to isoniazid. streptomycin and ethambutol (Abst.), *Am. Rev. Respir. Dis., 113, No. 4, Part 2:*65 (1976).

385. Tsukamura, M., Grouping of mycobacteria by means of utilization of inorganic nitrogen source (in Japanese with English abst.), *Med. Biol. 71:*286–289 (1965).

386. Tsukamura, M., Identification of mycobacteria, *Tubercle 48:*311–338 (1967).

387. Tsukamura, M., Relationship between the growth rate of mycobacteria and their ability to utilize organic acids as the sole source of carbon, *Jap. J. Microbiol. 12:*534–536 (1968).

388. Tsukamura, M., Identification of Group II scotochromogens and Group III nonphotochromogens of mycobacteria, *Tubercle 50:*51–60 (1969).

389. Tsukamura, M., Differentiation between *Mycobacterium abscessus* and Mycobacterium borstelense, Am. Rev. Respir. Dis., 101:426–428 (1970).

390. Tsukamura, M., Susceptibility of *Mycobacterium intracellulare* to rifampicin: A trial of ecological observation, *Jap. J. Microbiol. 16:*444–446 (1972).

391. Tsukamura, M., Roentgenographic features of lung disease due to *Mycobacterium intracellulare* (primary and secondary infection), *Kekkaku* (author's summary in Engl.) *50:*17–30 (1975).

392. Tsukamura, M., and Mizuno, S., "Hypothetical mean organisms of Mycobacteria," A study of classification of mycobacteria, *Jap. J. Microbiol. 12:*371–384 (1968).

393. Tsukamura, M., Mizuno, S., Murata, H., Nemoto, H., and Yugi, H., A comparative study of mycobacteria from patients' room dusts and from sputa of tuberculous patients, *Jap. J. Microbiol. 18:*271–277 (1974).

394. Tsukamura, M., Nakamura, E., Kurita, I., and Nakamura, T., Isolation of *Mycobacterium chelonei,* subspecies *chelonei, (Mycobacterium borstelense)* from pulmonary lesions of 9 patients, *Am. Rev. Respir. Dis., 108:*683–685 (1973).

395. Tsukamura, M., and Nemoto, H., A taxonomic study of *Mycobacterium intracellulare* isolated from swine, *Jap. J. Microbiol. 17:*91–98 (1973).

396. Tsukamura, M., *et al.* (sic), Differentiation of *Mycobacterium avium* and *M. intracellulare* by utilization of butanol as carbon source: Comparison of Japanese and United States isolates of *M. intracellulare, Kekkaku 46:*197–202 (1971). Abst. in *Am. Rev. Respir. Dis. 105:*169 (1972).

397. Tsukamura, M., Shimoide, H., Kita, N., Segawa, J., Ito, T., Kondo, H., Shirota, N., Tamura, M., Matsuda, N., Kuse, A., and Yamamoto, Y., A study on the frequency of "atypical" mycobacteria and "atypical" mycobacteriosis in Japanese National Hospitals, *Kekkaku 48:*203–211 (1973).

398. Tsukamura, M., Shimoide, H., Segawa, I., Kita, N., Shirota, N., Kondo, H., Tamura, M., Ito, T., Kuse, A., Matsuda, N., and Yamamoto, Y., Clinical features of lung disease due to *Mycobacterium intracellulare, Kekakku, 49:*139–145 (1974).

399. Tsukamura, M., Toyama, H., and Tsukamura, S., A comparative study of the virulence for mice in "atypical" and named mycobacteria from human and soil sources, *Jap. J. Tuberc. 13:*49–64 (1966).

400. Tsukamura, M., and Tsukamura, S., Differentiation of *Mycobacterium tuberculosis*

and *Mycobacterium bovis* by *p*-nitrobenzoic acid susceptibility, *Tubercle 45:*64–65 (1964).

401. Tsukamura, M., and Tsukamura, S., A practical system for identification of *Mycobacterium tuberculosis, Mycobacterium bovis, Mycobacterium kansasii,* and *Mycobacterium fortuitum, Scand. J. Respir. Dis. 48:*58–70 (1967).

402. Tsukamura, M., and Tsukamura, S., Further observations on *Mycobacterium terrae, Am. Rev. Respir. Dis. 96:*299–304 (1967).

403. Tsukamura, M., Tsukamura, S., Mizuno, S., and Toyama, H., Bacteriological studies on atypical mycobacteria isolated in Japan. Report III. A comparison between pathogenic scotochromogens and soil scotochromogens, *Kekkaku 42:*15–21 (1967).

404. van der Hoeven, L. H., Rutten, F. J., and Van der Sar, A., An unusual acid-fast bacillus causing systemic disease and death in a child, *Am. J. Clin. Pathol. 29:*433–448 (1958).

405. Van Dyke, J. J., and Lake, K. B., Chemotherapy for aquarium granuloma, *J. Amer. Med. Assoc. 233:*1380–1381 (1975).

406. Van Zeben, W., Lymphadenitis tuberculose scrofulacea, *Maandschr. Kindergeneeskd.* (Abst.–Sum. in Eng.) *22:*393–401 (1959).

407. Van Zeben, W., Tuberculosis in children caused by "atypical" mycobacteria, *R. Neth. Tuberc. Assoc. Selected Papers 7:*61–71 (1963).

408. Virtanen, S., A study of the nitrate reduction by mycobacteria. The use of the nitrate reduction test in the identification of mycobacteria, *Acta Tuberc. Scand. 1960, Suppl. 48:*1–119.

409. Virtanen, S., Drug sensitivities of atypical acid-fast organisms, *Acta Tuberc. Scand. 40:*182–189 (1961).

410. Virtanen, S., On the importance of atypical acid-fast organisms as pathogenic agents, *Acta Tuberc. Scand. 40:*190–194 (1961).

411. Volini, F., Colton, R., and Lester, W., Disseminated infection caused by Battey type mycobacteria, *Am. J. Clin. Pathol. 43:*39–46 (1965).

412. Walker, H. H., Shinn, M. F., Higaki, M., and Ogata, J., Some characteristics of "swimming pool" disease in Hawaii, *Hawaii Med. J. 21:*403–409 (1962).

413. Ward, A. R., Die Invasion des Eyters durch Bakterien, *Zentralbl. Bakteriol. Parasitenkd. Infectionskr. Hyg. Abt. 1 Orig. 27:*680 (1900). (Abst. from Bull. 178, Cornell University Agricultural Experiment Station.)

414. Warring, F. C., Jr., Mycobacteria in a New England Hospital: A study of mycobacterial species in the sputum of patients with chronic pulmonary disease, *Am. Rev. Respir. Dis. 98:*965–977 (1968).

415. Wassermann, H. E., Avian tuberculous endophthalmitis, *Arch. Ophthalmol. 89:*321–323 (1973).

416. Watanakunakorn, C., and Trott, A., Vertebral osteomyelitis due to *Mycobacterium kansasii, Am. Rev. Respir. Dis. 107:*846–850 (1973).

417. Wayne, L. G., The mycobacterial mystique: Deterrent to taxonomy, *Am. Rev. Respir. Dis. 90:*255–257 (1964).

418. Wayne, L. G., Classification and identification of mycobacteria: III. Species within Group III, *Am. Rev. Respir. Dis. 93:*918–928 (1966).

419. Wayne, L. G., and Doubek, J. R., The role of air in the photochromogenic behavior of *Mycobacterium kansasii, Am. J. Clin. Pathol. 42:*431–433 (1964).

420. Wayne, L. G., and Doubek, J. R., Classification and identification of mycobacteria. II.

Tests employing nitrate and nitrite as substrate, *Am. Rev. Respir. Dis. 91:*738–745 (1965).

421. Wayne, L. G., Doubek, J. R., and Russell, R. L., Classification and identification of mycobacteria. I. Tests employing Tween 80 as substrate, *Am. Rev. Respir. Dis. 90:*588–597 (1964).

422. Weed, L. A., Karlson, A. G., Ivins, J. C., and Miller, R. H., Recurring migratory chronic osteomyelitis associated with saprophytic acid-fast bacilli: Report of a case of 10 years' duration apparently cured by surgery, *Proc. Staff Meetings Mayo Clin. 31:*238–246 (1956).

423. Weed, L. A., Keith, H. M., and Needham, G. M., Non-tuberculous acid-fast cervical adenitis in children, *Proc. Staff Meetings Mayo Clin. 31:*259–263 (1956).

424. Weed, L. A., McDonald, J. R., and Needham, G. M., The isolation of "saprophytic" acid-fast bacilli from lesions of caseous granulomas, *Proc. Staff Meetings Mayo Clin. 31:*246–258 (1956).

425. Weiszfeiler, G., *et al.* (sic), Two new facultative pathogenic mycobacterium species named *M. simiae* and *M. asiaticum, Tuberkulosiz 10:*289–293 (1973). Abst. in *Am. Rev. Respir. Dis. 106:*158 (1972).

426. Wenkle, W. C., Loomis, R. N., and Jarboe, J. M., Chromogenic acid-fast bacilli, *Am. Rev. Tuberc. Pulm. Dis. 57:*385–388 (1948).

427. Wichelhausen, R. H., and Robinson, L. B., Further studies in classification, growth characteristics and drug susceptibility determinations in mycobacteria other than *M. tuberculosis, Transactions of the 25th Research Conference in Pulmonary Disease,* pp. 71–79 (1966).

428. Wijsmuller, G., and Erickson, P., The reaction to PPD-Battey. A new look, *Am. Rev. Respir. Dis. 109:*29–40 (1974).

429. Wijsmuller, G., Narain, R., Mayurnath, S., and Palmer, C. E., On the nature of tuberculin sensitivity in South India, *Am. Rev. Respir. Dis. 97:*429–443 (1968).

430. Williston, E. H., and Youmans, G. P., Streptomycin-resistant strains of tubercle bacilli, *Am. Rev. Tuberc. Pulm. Dis. 55:*536–539 (1947).

431. Wolinsky, E., Experience with atypical mycobacterial infections in man, *in* "The Anonymous Mycobacteria in Human Disease" (J. S. Chapman, Ed.), pp. 45–51, Charles C Thomas, Springfield, Ill. (1960).

432. Wolinsky, E., Experimental chemotherapy of atypical mycobacterial infection, *in* "The Anonymous Mycobacteria in Human Disease" (J. S. Chapman, Ed.), pp. 132–144, Charles C Thomas, Springfield, Ill. (1960).

433. Wolinsky, E., The role of the scotochromogenic mycobacteria in human disease, *Ann. N.Y. Acad. Sci. 106:*67–71 (1963).

434. Wolinsky, E., Gomez, F., and Zimpfer, F., Sporotrichoid *Mycobacterium marinum* infection treated with rifampin–ethambutol, *Am. Rev. Respir. Dis. 105:*964–967 (1972).

435. Wood, L. E., Buhler, V. B., and Pollak, A., Human infection with the "yellow" acid-fast bacillus. A report of fifteen additional cases, *Am. Rev. Tuberc. Pulm. Dis. 73:*917–929 (1956).

436. Worthington, R. W., and Kleeberg, H. H., Isolation of *Mycobacterium kansasii* from bovines, *S. Afr. Vet. Med. Assoc. 35:*29–33 (1964).

437. Wright, G. L., Jr., and Roberts, D. B., Two-dimensional electrophoresis of mycobacterial antigens: Comparison with a reference system, *Am. Rev. Respir. Dis. 109:*306–310 (1974).

438. Wunsh, S. E., Boyle, G. L., Leopold, I. H., and Littman, M. L., *Mycobacterium fortuitum* infection of corneal graft, *Arch. Ophthalmol. 82:*602–607 (1969).

439. Xalabardier, C., The so-called problem of unclassified mycobacteria, *Am. Rev. Respir. Dis. 83:*1–15 (1961).

440. Yakovac, W. C., Baker, R., Sweigert, C., and Hope, J. W., Fatal disseminated osteomyelitis due to an anonymous mycobacterium, *Pediatrics 59:*909–914 (1961).

441. Yamamoto, M., Ogura, Y., Sudo, K., and Hibino, S., Diagnostic criteria for disease caused by atypical mycobacteria, *Am. Rev. Respir. Dis. 96:*773–778 (1967).

442. Yamamoto, M., Sudo, K., Taga, M., and Hibino, S., A study of disease caused by atypical mycobacteria in Japan, *Am. Rev. Respir. Dis. 96:*779–787 (1967).

443. Yeager, H., Jr., and Raleigh, J. W., Pulmonary disease due to *Mycobacterium intracellulare, Am. Rev. Respir. Dis. 108:*547–552 (1973).

444. Yoder, W. D., and Schaefer, W. B., Comparison of the sero-agglutination test with the pathogenicity test in the chicken for the identification of *Mycobacterium avium* and *Mycobacterium intracellulare, Am. Rev. Respir. Dis. 103:*173–178 (1971).

445. Yue, W. Y., and Cohen, S. S., Pulmonary infection caused by niacin-positive *Mycobacterium kansasii, Am. Rev. Respir. Dis. 94:*447–449 (1966).

446. Zak, F., and Sula, L., Experimental studies in the morphology of vole bacillus infection in cattle, with a contribution to the development of the so-called Schaumann bodies, *Pathol. Microbiol. 23:*456–471 (1960).

447. Zamorano, J., Jr., and Tompsett, R., Disseminated atypical mycobacterial infection and pancytopenia, *Arch Intern. Med. 121:*424–427 (1968).

448. Zimmerman, L. E., Turner, L., and McTigue, J. W., *Mycobacterium fortuitum* infection of the cornea. A report of two cases, *Arch. Ophthalmol. 82:*596–601 (1969).

449. Zvetina, J. R., Clinical characteristics of pulmonary infection associated with *M. kansasii, Transactions of the 25th Research Conference in Pulmonary Disease,* pp. 79–83 (1966).

REPORTS OF COMMITTEES AND SUBCOMMITTEES

450. Subcommittee on Mycobacteria, American Society for Microbiology, *Mycobacterium kansasii* (Hauduroy), *J. Bacteriol. 83:*931–932 (1962).

451. A report from the Research Committee of the British Tuberculosis Association, *Tubercle 47:*157–177 (1966).

452. The Cooperative Study Group of the Japanese National Study Group on Atypical Mycobacteria, A study of "atypical" mycobacteria in Japanese National Sanatoria, *Tubercle 51:*270–279 (1970).

453. The Cooperative Study Group of the National Sanatoriums on Atypical Mycobacteria, A study on the frequency of atypical mycobacterial infections in Japanese National Sanatoriums, *Jap. J. Tuberc. Chest Dis. 30:*119–127 (1971). Abst. in *Am. Rev. Respir. Dis. 104:*152 (1971).

Index

191